MW00843461

For access to digital chapters, visit the APHA Press bookstore (www.apha.org).

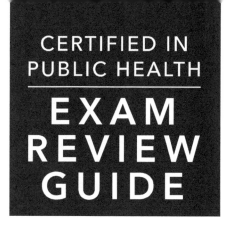

CERTIFIED IN PUBLIC HEALTH

EXAM REVIEW GUIDE

editors
Karen D. Liller, PhD, CPH
Jaime A. Corvin, PhD, MSPH, CPH

associate editor
Hari H. Venkatachalam, MPH, CPH

American Public Health Association
800 I Street, NW
Washington, DC 20001-3710
www.apha.org

Georges Benjamin, MD, Executive Director

Printed and bound in the United States of America
Book Production Editor: Maya Ribault
Typesetting: The Charlesworth Group
Cover Design: Alan Giarcanella
Printing and Binding: Sheridan Books

Library of Congress Cataloging-in-Publication Data

Names: Liller, Karen DeSafey, editor. | Corvin, Jaime A., editor. |
     Venkatachalam, Hari H., editor. | American Public Health Association,
     issuing body.
Title: Certified in public health : exam review guide / editors, Karen D.
     Liller and Jaime A. Corvin ; associate editor, Hari H. Venkatachalam.
Description: Washington, DC : American Public Health Association, [2018] |
     Includes bibliographical references.
Identifiers: LCCN 2018043626 (print) | LCCN 2018044316 (ebook) | ISBN
     9780875532981 (ebook) | ISBN 9780875532974 (softcover)
Subjects: | MESH: Public Health | Outlines | Examination Questions
Classification: LCC RA425 (ebook) | LCC RA425 (print) | NLM WA 18.2 | DDC
     362.1--dc23
LC record available at https://lccn.loc.gov/2018043626

Contents

Preface

As editors, we are excited to bring you this review guide to help prepare you for certification in public health. It is our hope that this book will help you successfully prepare for the Certified in Public Health (CPH) exam administered by the National Board of Public Health Examiners (NBPHE) and aid in your professional advancement.

You may be asking yourself, Why should I get certified? The NBPHE Web site (https://www.nbphe.org/why-get-certified) reminds us that the benefits of being CPH-certified are many. Benefits include staying current on best practices and education, meeting and maintaining a national professional standard, gaining increased recognition in the public health professions, investing in your career, evidence of mastery of the public health sciences, potential for promotion and salary increases, distinguishing yourself from peers, going beyond your education, and raising the visibility of public health. Through this process, you are embarking on a journey, one that is helping to professionalize the CPH degree and has resulted in a cadre of public health professionals poised to address 21st century public health challenges.

Each chapter in this text is built around the new domains and tasks in public health that were developed by NBPHE from a broad-based job task analysis and focus on integration of major concepts that reflect the real world of public health. Chapters cover the following topics: evidence-based approaches to public health, communication, leadership, law and ethics, biological determinants of health, collaboration and partnership, program planning and evaluation, program management, policy in public health, and health equity and social justice. Within each chapter, you will see the associated job tasks and a review of the major critical content. Beside tasks, you will note checkboxes that you can mark complete once you feel you have a full understanding of the tasks and related concepts. You will also find case studies and/or shorter vignettes or questions in each chapter to allow you to put your knowledge into practice. In addition, references are provided to add to your understanding.

The editors and authors of this guide—all faculty at the University of South Florida College of Public Health(USF COPH)—are deeply committed to the advancement of public health. These authors have worked together to develop and teach an integrated core curriculum for all master's students in the College, one designed to better address the interdisciplinary, dynamic, and changing world of public health. The authors also served as the review guide's advisory committee in the development of this text.

The editors would like to acknowledge the chapter authors for their hard work, as well as the leadership, faculty, staff, and students of USF COPH whose support of and dedication to public health are unparalleled. We would like to especially acknowledge Evan Hegarty and other USF COPH students who reviewed text chapters for quality and Carlos Montoya for his exemplary drawings of several text figures. Finally, we wish to thank the American Public Health Association Press for their support and guidance throughout the publication of this text.

We extend our best wishes for your success with a message from Allison Foster, MBA, CAE, President of NBPHE:

> On behalf of the National Board of Public Health Examiners, we applaud your decision to pursue Certification in Public Health which will advance both your career and the field of public health. In conjunction with your educational and work experiences, and other study resources, this review book will be a useful tool in preparation for taking the CPH examination. Good luck in your pursuit of certification!

Karen D. Liller, PhD, CPH
Jaime A. Corvin, PhD, MSPH, CPH
Hari H. Venkatachalam, MPH, CPH

Evidence-Based Approaches to Public Health

Janice Zgibor, PhD, Chighaf Bakour, MD, PhD, CPH, Wei Wang, PhD,
Kathleen O'Rourke, PhD, CPH, Troy Quast, PhD, and
Hari H. Venkatachalam, MPH, CPH

A. Concepts of Epidemiology

INTRODUCTION

This chapter is divided into two sections and will review evidence-based approaches to public health. The focus of Section A of this chapter is the epidemiologic concepts that will be critical to your success as a public health professional. Several biostatistical concepts are introduced in this portion, and these concepts are further developed in Section B. This chapter contains many diagrams based on concepts and formulas widely found throughout the literature to help aid in your understanding.

According to Brownson et al., "Evidence-based public health is defined as the development, implementation, and evaluation of effective programs and policies in public health through application of principles of scientific reasoning, including systematic uses of data and information systems, and appropriate use of behavioral science theory and program planning models."[1] Although this definition is very broad, the methods used to develop public health programs and evaluation of these programs are specific.

Why do we care about using evidence-based approaches in public health? We need to know that decision-making is based on scientific evidence and that interventions that have been shown to be effective are implemented. Evidence-based public health approaches ensure that we have reliable information so that we can be more confident that we are implementing the best practices. This evidence base is also important when one is evaluating effectiveness and costs when implementing new health programs, establishing new policies, and conducting literature reviews. Generating the evidence for public health practice is often transdisciplinary, which means teams of researchers from a variety of disciplines contribute to the evidence base.[1,2]

In our analysis of evidence-based approaches, we will first review common terminology that is used in scientific evidence produced for dissemination in the literature or by the public. Next, we will review some of the basic calculations used in research studies. Finally, we will review the importance of surveillance systems and data sets.

After studying this chapter, you should be able to perform the following tasks:

❑ Interpret results of statistical analyses found in public health studies or reports.
❑ Interpret quantitative or qualitative data following current scientific standards.
❑ Apply common statistical methods for inference.
❑ Apply descriptive techniques commonly used to summarize public data.
❑ Identify the limitations of research results, data sources, or existing practices and programs.
❑ Use statistical packages or software to analyze data.
❑ Synthesize information from multiple data systems or other sources.
❑ Identify key sources of data for epidemiologic or other public health investigation purposes.
❑ Calculate mortality, morbidity, and health risk factor rates.
❑ Collect valid and reliable quantitative or qualitative data.
❑ Use information technology for data collection, storage, and retrieval.
❑ Illustrate how gender, race, ethnicity, and other evolving demographics affect the health of a population.
❑ Use population health surveillance systems.

MAJOR CONTENT

Common Epidemiologic Terms

Measures of Disease Frequency

Frequency measures are often used in epidemiology to characterize disease and risk occurrence in populations. Frequency measures share a common trait of being represented as fractions, and, therefore, all have a numerator and a denominator. The following are common types of disease frequency measures[3]:

- **Ratio**: Ratios are calculated by dividing one number by another. Unlike proportions, the numerator does not need to be a subset of the denominator as they are two distinct quantities (e.g., the ratio of men to women).
- **Proportion:** Proportions are calculated by dividing one number by another, where the numerator is a subset of the denominator (e.g., the proportion of men in a population calculated as the number of men divided by the total population).
- **Rate:** Similar to ratios and proportions, rates are calculated by dividing one number by another, and additionally have a time component as a part of the denominator (e.g., the number of people who developed influenza in 2017, the birth rate per year in a population, the mortality rate per year in a population).

Incidence and Prevalence

When one is assessing the disease burden in a population, two different types of measures can be used: **incidence** and **prevalence**. Both reveal different information, with incidence focusing on occurrence of new cases and prevalence being a measure of existing cases in a population:

1. **Incidence:** A measure of the number of new cases of a disease. Pre-existing cases of the disease are not counted. Incidence can be assessed as a proportion, in the form of "cumulative incidence," or as a rate, in the form of "incidence rate."
   a. **Cumulative incidence**: The number of new cases of disease in a population over a specified time period.
   b. **Incidence rate:** The number of new cases of the disease during person-time of observation. Time is measured as the amount of time people are followed or exposed ranging from before the onset of disease to the end of follow-up.
2. **Prevalence**: The number of existing cases of a disease during a given time period. This includes cases that already existed as well as new cases that developed during the time.
   a. **Point prevalence:** The proportion of the population that is diseased at a single point in time (a calendar date, a point in life such as college graduation).[4]
   b. **Period prevalence:** The proportion of the population that is diseased during a specific duration of time, such as a year.

Disease Distribution Terms

Epidemiologic investigations of outbreaks of diseases warrant the need for describing situations in which disease rates are elevated. Common terms include the following:

- **Endemic:** A situation in a community in which there is a consistent elevated rate of a certain disease.
- **Epidemic:** An increase in the number of cases of disease in a community, above what is expected.
- **Pandemic:** A worldwide epidemic.

Overview of Study Designs

The evidence base of public health is built through research that uses a variety of study designs. When researchers have a specific hypothesis to test, they must determine the best study design to use. There are two overall types of epidemiologic study designs: **descriptive** and **analytic**. Descriptive studies are generally observational, whereas analytic studies can be both interventional (experimental) and observational (see Figure 1-1). Different designs work better in different situations at different points along the research continuum.

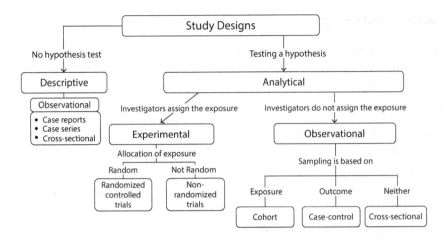

Figure 1-1. Type of Study Designs

As we will see, the types of study also differ on what characteristics we use to enroll people into the study. Descriptions of types of studies (this does not include expert opinions) are as follows:

1. Types of descriptive studies:
   a. **Case studies** and **case reports**: Studies used to alert people of a new illness or new association with illness. They usually are reports of only people with the condition of interest.
   b. **Cross-sectional studies**: Studies that include people who are representative of a given population. They are not selected on the basis of illness or exposure and can be used to determine initial associations and to identify the prevalence of either exposure or illness in a group.
   c. **Ecological studies**: Studies that are used to describe populations. The data are not analyzed on the individual level, but rather on the aggregate level. These studies may suffer from the **ecological fallacy.** The ecological fallacy occurs when group-level data are used to report on individuals.
2. Types of analytic studies:
   a. **Case–control studies**: Studies that select people with or without disease and then proceed to look back over time to see if people had different rates of exposure. Case–control studies are good for rare diseases with long **latency periods**. A long latency period refers to diseases that take a long time to develop. For example, many cancers have a long latency period.
   b. **Cohort studies**: Studies that select people on the basis of exposure and determine if people develop disease at different rates. Cohort studies are good for rare exposures and may follow individuals into the future (**prospective**) or look back in time

(**retrospective**). Incidence can be calculated from such studies. People who have disease at the time point when the study period begins (**prevalence cases**) are excluded.

c. **Randomized controlled trials (RCT):** RCTs test an intervention that is given by the researcher to two or more groups. People are randomly assigned into groups (**randomization**), and some are given the active item (e.g., medicine, diet, educational program) while the other group(s) are given the usual treatment, nothing, or a **placebo**. The researcher then follows the resulting treatment groups over time and compares outcomes between the groups to determine the effects of the intervention. Research participants often do not know which group they are in, and at times researchers also do not know who is getting which treatment (**single** and **double blinding,** respectively).

d. **Systematic reviews and meta-analyses:** These are studies that pool the results of multiple independent studies with established criteria to identify the evidence for associations.

Studies can be ordered in a hierarchical manner by the amount of evidence they provide for epidemiologic associations from the lowest to the highest amount of evidence. In Figure 1-2, expert opinion is the lowest level and systematic reviews are the highest level of evidence.

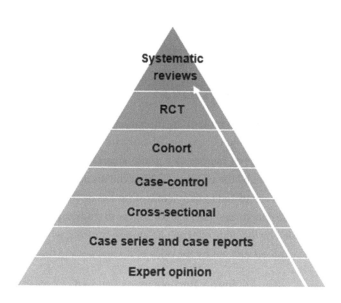

Note: RCT = randomized controlled trial.

Figure 1-2. Hierarchy of Types of Study Designs by Amount of Evidence Collected

Table 1-1. Example of a 2 × 2 Table for Epidemiological Calculations

	Outcome	No Outcome	Total
Exposure	A	B	A + B
No Exposure	C	D	C + D
Total	A + C	B + D	A + B + C + D

Epidemiologic Calculations

Measures of Association: 2 × 2 Tables

An association between an exposure and an outcome is usually calculated in public health research with various epidemiologic measures. To perform these calculations, epidemiologists often consolidate their data into 2 × 2 tables (see Table 1-1). From the values input into the cells of the 2 × 2 table, various measures of association can be calculated.

Measures of Association: Relative Risk

Relative risk (RR) is a measure of the magnitude of an association between an exposure and a disease that is used in cohort studies. It is a ratio of the risk (incidence) of disease in the exposed to the risk in the nonexposed:

$$RR = \frac{\text{Risk (Incidence) of Outcome in the Exposed}}{\text{Risk (Incidence) of Outcome in the Nonexposed}}$$

$$= \frac{A/(A + B)}{C/(C + D)}$$

Measures of Association: Odds Ratio

The odds of an event occurring is a ratio of the probability of the event occurring divided by the probability of the event not occurring. This is often expressed as the formula of $p/(1-p)$. For example, the odds of disease in a group are calculated as the number with the disease of interest divided by the number without the disease of interest.

The **odds ratio (OR)** is calculated in case–control studies or cross-sectional studies, as we do not have incidence data to calculate the RR for those studies. It is the odds of exposure among cases divided by the odds of exposure among controls, which equals the odds of disease among the exposed divided by the odds of disease among the nonexposed:

$$OR = \frac{\text{Odds of Outcome in the Exposed}}{\text{Odds of Outcome in the Nonexposed}}$$

$$= \frac{A/B}{C/D} = \frac{AD}{BC}$$

Interpretation of Measures of Association

The values calculated from the measures of association can help inform public health professionals about the correlation between the exposure and the outcome. It should be noted that these values first inform on **correlation** and not **causation.** Secondly, the correlation is only relevant to the specific tested sample, and such results may not be the same in the larger population. Finally, these associations can be susceptible to various forms of bias, misclassification, and random error. Therefore, researchers need to be careful when interpreting the results from these measures of association not to make broad generalizations, but to always analyze the data with scrutiny. The following provides guidance for interpreting measures of association:

- RR or OR = 1: Means there is no association between the exposure and outcome. The risk or odds in the exposed equals the risk or odds in the nonexposed.
- RR or OR > 1: Means the exposure increases the risk of the outcome. The risk or odds in the exposed is greater than the risk or odds in the nonexposed.
- RR or OR < 1: Means the exposure decreases the risk of the outcome. The risk or odds in the exposed is less than the risk or odds in the nonexposed. This indicates that the exposure is a **protective factor.**

Example of Relative Risk Calculation:

	Asthma	No Asthma	Total
Smoker	60	140	200
Nonsmoker	80	720	800
Total	140	860	1,000

Calculate the incidence of asthma in smokers (exposed)	= 60/200 = 0.3 (30%)
Calculate the incidence of asthma in nonsmokers (nonexposed)	= 80/800 = 0.1 (10%)
Calculate the relative risk	= 0.3/0.1 = 3

Interpretation: Smokers have three times the risk of asthma as nonsmokers. Smoking increases the risk of asthma by 3 times.

Example of Odds Ratio Calculation:

	Liver Cancer	No Liver Cancer	Total
Diabetes	25	15	40
No diabetes	275	585	860
Total	300	600	900

Calculate the odds ratio	= (25 × 585) / (15 × 275) = 3.55

Interpretation: The odds of having diabetes are **3.55** times higher in people with liver cancer compared with those without liver cancer.

Or: The odds of having liver cancer are **3.55** times higher in people with diabetes compared with those without diabetes.

Errors in Epidemiology

When one identifies associations between an exposure and an outcome, there are potential errors that can occur. There are three reasons why epidemiologists may obtain a false association between an exposure and an outcome from sample data. First, the finding can be attributable to chance alone—just the luck of the draw. Second, there could be some **bias** in the study methodology that led to the incorrect finding. Finally, there may be some **confounding** from another variable.

Bias

Bias is a systematic error as compared to an error attributable to chance alone. Bias can cause an error in the estimation of an association between an exposure and an outcome. This error can act in different ways:

- The bias can cause us to believe there is an association when there is none, or **bias away from the null**.
- The bias can hide an association that actually exists, or **bias toward the null**.

Bias can occur in the design phase and/or during the conduct of the study. One can evaluate bias during the analysis and identify its potential effect, but it cannot be fixed at that time. Researchers can introduce bias as they make decisions as to how data are being collected or how people are selected into study groups. Furthermore, participants themselves can introduce bias.

There are two main types of bias:

1. **Selection bias**: This bias results from procedures used to select participants into a study. Such bias would result in a different outcome from what would have been obtained from the entire population targeted for the study. This bias most likely occurs in case–control or retrospective cohort studies because the exposure and outcome have occurred at the time of study selection. Selection bias can also occur in prospective cohort studies and experimental studies from differential loss to follow-up because this affects which subjects are "selected" for analysis.

2. **Observation bias**: This bias arises from systematic differences in the way information on exposure or disease is obtained from the study groups. It is also known as **information bias**. Observation bias occurs only after the participants have entered the study. There are several types of observation bias. These include **recall bias** (inaccurate reporting of past events), **interviewer bias** (may include the effects of the interviewer's body language, voice, or demeanor on the response; it is the most difficult bias to account for), and **misclassification. Misclassification error** happens when participants are incorrectly classified into the wrong population, distorting the link between exposure and outcome. It can result from participants being incorrectly classified as either exposed or unexposed or having the outcome or not having the

outcome. Misclassification may be **differential** (bias is different between groups) and **nondifferential** (bias is equal across groups).

Confounding

Confounding occurs when a researcher is evaluating the relationship between an exposure and an outcome, but a third variable, which is associated with both the exposure and the outcome, distorts the finding. A confounder cannot be on the causal pathway between the exposure and the outcome. A confounder can create a bias toward the null or away from the null. There are several ways to prevent confounding and also to manage confounding during the analysis stage. These methods are **randomization**, **restriction**, **matching**, **standardization**, **stratification**, and conducting a **multivariable analysis**.

Effect Modification

Effect modification occurs when the magnitude of the association between an exposure and outcome varies by the presence or level of a third variable. For example, we know that smokers who are exposed to asbestos have a much higher rate of lung cancer than smokers without asbestos exposure.

Confounding Versus Effect Modification

What is the difference between a confounder and an effect modifier? They both are a third variable that has an impact on the association between the exposure and the outcome. A confounder, however, distorts the true association. It can incorrectly make the association appear stronger or weaker than it really is. By contrast, an effect modifier actually clarifies the association. It provides us with more information than we would have had otherwise. When one conducts the analysis, one needs to control for the impact of a confounder, but to evaluate for the impact of an effect modifier.

It is important to recognize that a variable can be a confounder, an effect modifier, or both at the same time. Differentiating among whether a variable is one, the other, or both can be done through **stratification** by the variable. Stratification divides the data according to the levels of the variable and allows the calculation of a measure of association for each strata (see Table 1-2).

The obtained measures of association from a stratified analysis can be used to assess confounding and effect modification:

- If the variable is only a confounder, stratum-specific estimates for the measure of association, either the OR or RR, will be close to one another. The **crude**, or overall, estimate will be outside the range of the stratum-specific estimates. In other words, the crude estimate will be either greater than all the stratum-specific estimates or less than all estimates.

Table 1-2. Stratified Data Sets for Assessment of Effect Modification and Confounding

Data Set	Crude RR	Stratum 1 RR	Stratum 2 RR	Is There Evidence of Effect Modification?	Is There Evidence of Confounding?
1	2.10	1.10	3.10	Yes	No
2	5.20	1.40	1.30	No	Yes
3	1.30	3.20	7.50	Yes	Yes
4	3.10	3.20	3.00	No	No

Note: RR=relative risk.

- If the variable is only an effect modifier, the stratum-specific estimates for the OR and the RR will be significantly different from one another. The crude estimate will be within the range of all the stratum-specific estimates.
- If the variable is both a confounder and an effect modifier, stratum-specific estimates for the OR or RR will be significantly different from one another. Also, the crude estimate will be considerably outside the range of stratum-specific estimates.

Causation

One reason identifying causation is so difficult is that it can be hard to identify the difference between correlation and causation. There are a number of models used to explore this. One of the early criteria to identify causation was **Koch's postulates.** Koch's postulates were generally more effective for determining the causative agent for infectious disease. These postulates are as follows[5]:

- The microorganism must be found in abundance in all organisms suffering from the disease, but should not be found in healthy organisms.
- It should be possible to isolate the causative microorganism from a diseased organism and grow it in pure culture.
- The organism from pure culture should be able to cause disease when inoculated into a healthy host organism.
- The microorganism should then be able to be isolated from the new host and grown in pure culture.

A newer model of causation was developed in 1965 by Sir Bradford Hill, which expanded on previous concepts. **Hill's Nine Criteria of Causality** proved to be more effective in evaluating chronic disease. The more criteria that an association met, the more likely it was that there was a causal association between an exposure and an outcome[6]:

1. **Analogy**: When a researcher can identify a similar relationship between another exposure and/or disease. It provides evidence for a biological pathway that might be due to causation.

2. **Coherence**: Considers the entire picture of the association between an exposure and outcome across different models.
3. **Reversibility**: Considers if removing the exposure diminishes the probability or occurrence of disease. If an individual is no longer exposed, does his or her disease diminish?
4. **Specificity**: Specificity indicates that one exposure should cause one disease. It is more relevant to infectious diseases, although it does not even always hold true there.
5. **Plausibility:** Refers to whether or not the exposure is likely to cause the disease. Is there a biological or social model that can explain the association? Does the association not conflict with current science?
6. **Strength of the association:** Refers to the fact that the stronger the association, the more likely it is attributable to a causal factor. This is because strong associations are less likely to totally result from bias and confounding. Chance is less likely to play a major role.
7. **Consistency:** Considers regularity of an association across multiple studies.
8. **Biological gradient**: A measure of the dose–response relationship. Does the risk of disease increase with the risk of exposure? Do higher levels of exposure cause higher levels of disease?
9. **Temporality**: Often considered the most important criteria. The exposure must come before the disease.

Levels of Prevention

Epidemiologists focus on prevention. The different levels of prevention depend on which stage of the natural history of a disease the prevention is targetting:

1. **Primordial prevention**: Earliest stage of prevention. It is concerned with preventing risk factors of disease by targeting lifestyles, behaviors, and exposure patterns at the aggregate level instead of the individual level in order to decrease the risk of disease. An example would include the enactment of policies that regulate calorie-dense foods to prevent obesity, a known risk factor for cardiovascular disease.
2. **Primary prevention**: Concerned with preventing disease. It takes place before the biological onset of disease. An example is having individuals use condoms so they do not acquire a sexually transmitted infection.
3. **Secondary prevention:** Prevention addressed by most screening programs. It occurs in the preclinical phase, after the disease is present but before symptoms appear. The focus is on early detection so that treatment can be provided before disease progresses. A classic example is annual screening for breast cancer with mammography.
4. **Tertiary prevention**: Focused on rehabilitation and support. As the disease has already occurred, the goal is to improve quality of life and reduce symptoms. An example would include patient education and support following diagnosis with diabetes.

Screening

Screening is a technique used to identify individuals who have a disease before symptoms occur with the goal of providing treatment before they experience any illness. Screening is conducted in the preclinical phase of the disease and is designed to be standardized across populations.[7]

An important characteristic of screening tests is determining **feasibility**. Feasibility is concerned with how likely the target audience is to participate in a recommended screening program. An example of a screening program with relatively low participation rates is that for colon cancer. According to the Centers for Disease Control and Prevention, about one in three adults aged 50 to 75 years have not been tested for colorectal cancer as recommended. This is attributable to the fact that the screening test is fairly invasive, the preparation for the screening is considered to be quite uncomfortable, and, in addition, there are sometimes cost-issue barriers. This is exemplified by the fact that about three quarters of those who were not screened did not have health insurance.[8]

Characteristics of Screening Tests

When evaluating a screening test for its usefulness, epidemiologists often consider the reliability and validity of the results. **Reliability** refers to repeatability. A reliable test is not necessarily valid. One can use a defective scale that underreports weight by 20 pounds each time. This scale is reliable, but it is not valid. Reliability is also depicted in the far-right image in Figure 1-3. In that image, the points are all clustered, showing how repeated measures were close to one another, but it still missed the bull's eye. Therefore, there is reliability, but not validity. The **validity** of a screening test is the ability of a test to accurately identify diseased and nondiseased individuals. As shown in the far-left image, the points are populated around the bull's eye, revealing increased validity. The lack of consistency in measurements, however, reveals poor reliability. The middle image in Figure 1-3 is a visual representation of valid and reliable measurements.

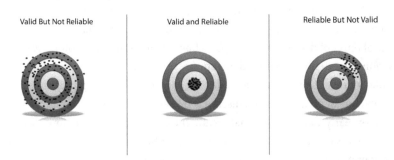

Valid But Not Reliable   Valid and Reliable   Reliable But Not Valid

Figure 1-3. Validity and Reliability

Validity of screening tests is measured by the sensitivity and specificity of the test. **Sensitivity** refers to the ability of a test to correctly identify the number of people with a disease. Those individuals who have the disease and who test positive for the disease are known as the **true positives**. Sensitivity is expressed as a percentage of those who truly have the disease. Therefore, the measure is a proportion in which the numerator is the true positives, while the denominator includes both the true positives and the individuals who have the disease but who do not test positive, called the **false negatives**. It is important to remember, though, that when we calculate sensitivity, we are only evaluating people with the disease.

By contrast, **specificity** refers to the ability of a test to correctly identify the number of people without a disease. Specificity is also expressed as a percentage, and it consists of a proportion. The numerator is those individuals who truly do not have the disease and test negative, or the **true negatives**. The denominator includes both the true negatives and those without the disease who tested positive, called the **false positives**. It is also, again, important to remember that when we calculate specificity, we are only evaluating people without the disease.

The **positive predictive value** of a screening test is also a proportion, for it is calculated as the number of people who test positive who actually have the disease divided by the number of positive tests. The difference between calculating the sensitivity and positive predictive value is, therefore, the denominator. Likewise, the **negative predictive value** is calculated as the number of people who test negative for a disease and do not have the disease divided by the total number of people who test negative. Again, the difference between the calculation of the negative predictive value and specificity is the denominator of the proportion.

Sensitivity, specificity, and negative and positive predictive values are determined by comparing the test to a **gold standard,** which is a definitive diagnosis that has been determined by biopsy, surgery, autopsy, or another method (see Table 1-3).

Table 1-3. Calculations[a] for Sensitivity, Specificity, Positive Predictive Value (PPV), and Negative Predictive Value (NPV)

		Gold Standard		
		Disease/condition present	Disease/condition absent	
Screening test results	Test + (T+)	A (true positives; TP)	B (false positives; FP)	Total T+
	Test − (T−)	C (false negatives; FN)	D (true negatives; TN)	Total T−
		Total with disease (D+)	Total without disease (D−)	

[a]NPV = D/(C + D) = [TN/total T−]; PPV = A/(A + B) = [TP/total T+]; sensitivity = A/(A + C) = TP/Total D+ = TP/(TP + FN); = TP/(TP + FN); specificity = D/(B + D) = TN/total D− = TN/(FP + TN).

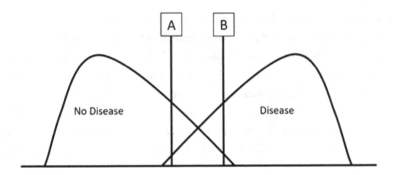

Notes: A and B are cutoff points that may be adjusted from center to maximize sensitivity and specificity.

Figure 1-4. Trade-Off Between Sensitivity and Specificity

Trade-Off Between Sensitivity and Specificity

Public health professionals desire to maximize both the sensitivity and specificity of a test. An ideal screening test would have a 100% sensitivity and 100% specificity or, in other words, have neither false negatives nor false positives. Screening tests, however, never achieve this level of validity. The cutoff point at which one determines that a screening test is positive or negative has an impact on both the specificity and sensitivity. As sensitivity and specificity are inversely related, adjustments to the cutoff necessitates a balancing of the need to maximize both sensitivity and specificity. If the cutoff value is set too low, the sensitivity of the screening test will be high but specificity will be low. On the other hand, if the cutoff value is set too high, specificity will increase, but sensitivity will decrease (see Figure 1-4).

Where a public health professional decides to make the cutoff depends on whether the greatest harm is in missing a disease or in falsely identifying a disease. A **receiver operating characteristic curve** (**ROC**) is used to set the cutoff value of a continuous value test. It shows the trade-off between sensitivity and specificity.

Screening tests are used to increase the life span of individuals screened by catching individuals with the disease before the development of symptoms and disease onset. This ability to increase the longevity of an individual may be exaggerated because of biases:

- **Lead time bias**: Overestimation of survival duration attributable to earlier detection by screening than by clinical presentation. Screening tests allow early detection and diagnosis of diseases. Individuals whose disease was identified through screening may appear to survive longer, even when the time from disease onset until death is similar to individuals whose disease was diagnosed later.
- **Length bias**: Screening is more likely to detect cases that are progressing slowly compared with those with rapid progression of disease, who manifest clinically. The slow-progressing cases are usually milder and more likely to survive, leading to an overestimation of survival as a result of screening.

Statistical Analysis, Surveillance, and Data Sets

Synthesizing Information From Multiple Data Systems or Other Sources

Often public health research includes data from multiple systems or sources. In these instances, it is imperative that researchers correctly synthesize the data sets across the sources. For instance, the researcher may need to merge data sets that are aggregated at different levels. It may be necessary to aggregate data at the zip code level to the county level, or the county level to the state level, or the state level to the national level. When doing so, researchers must carefully examine the variables to be aggregated. For count variables, simply adding the values across the subunits is appropriate. However, for variables that are averages or rates, the analyst must either sum up the values in the numerator and denominator then calculate the ratio or calculate a weighted average based on the denominator values.

Data sets may also differ in terms of the underlying collection methodologies, such as surveys, surveillance, or administrative data. Data sets may also contain differing variable types, including demographic, biometric, and attitudinal. The subject basis may also vary across data sets in which, for instance, the data could be a census, a simple sample, or a weighted sample. The underlying emphasis should be for the researcher to thoroughly investigate the structures of their data sets and variables and note how they differ. The researcher must then develop a plan to synthesize the data sets in a meaningful and appropriate way. It is imperative that any discussion of the resulting analysis includes a clear description of how the data sets were integrated.

Identifying Key Sources of Data for Epidemiologic or Other Public Health Investigation Purposes

Researchers today have many possible sources of data to study epidemiologic or public health topics. Often government sources are the most accessible and thorough. Examples of such data sets include the National Health and Nutrition Examination Survey, National Health Interview Survey, and the Behavioral Risk Factor Surveillance System. These data have typically been gathered to address a specific concern that may be aligned to a given research question. These data are usually viewed as being objective and reliable and many times are available on the Internet for download. Many governmental data series cover considerable time periods and allow for **longitudinal analyses**. When the governmental entity does not make a data set available online, researchers may be able to obtain the data via a data use agreement or **Freedom of Information Act** request.

There are many nongovernmental sources of research data. Community and nonprofit organizations often collect data on their activities and related impact. Think tanks may maintain internal and external data sets. There are also a number of commercial data sources from which researchers may obtain data. These data sets typically require payment and may involve a data use agreement in which the researcher agrees to only use the data for the specified purpose and to not share the data with others.

Interpreting Results of Statistical Analyses Found in Public Health Studies or Reports

Regardless of whether the individual is trying to operationalize previous studies or perform new research, it is critical that they correctly interpret the statistical analyses in public health studies. It is important for practitioners to be able to assess the quality of the statistical analysis of research and correctly interpret the magnitude of the estimates contained therein. Researchers must be able to assess the appropriateness of the approaches employed in the literature and determine whether a better option may be available. Often a key aspect of this assessment is to ascertain whether the modeling assumptions inherent in the given approach are likely to hold.

Assuming a study's estimation approach is valid, the interpretation of the findings of an inferential analysis can be summarized along two dimensions: **statistical significance** and **practical** (or **clinical**) **significance**. Statistical significance refers to whether the calculated estimate is likely to be observed assuming the null hypothesis of the test is true. *P*-values are measures of statistical significance in which lower values are associated with increased likelihood that the null hypothesis does not hold and are calculated based on formulas for a given inferential (see Section B of this chapter for more information on *p*-values and hypothesis testing). By contrast, practical significance is a subjective assessment of whether the effect estimated in a test is "important" or "meaningful." Unlike statistical significance, which is based on *p*-values, practical significance is typically not summarized in a specific measure. Instead, practical significance is based on the researcher's knowledge of the environment and judgment as to whether the estimated effect is meaningful.

Social Determinants of Health as a Basis for Social Epidemiology

The social determinants of health are factors in a social environment that contribute to or detract from the health of individuals and communities. These factors include but are not limited to the following: socioeconomic status, transportation, housing, access to services, discrimination by social grouping, and social or environmental stressors (see Chapter 10, "Health Equity and Social Justice," for more information on the social determinants of health).[9,10]

Surveillance

Surveillance is the systematic ongoing collection, analysis, interpretation, and dissemination of health data. Examples of US surveillance systems include those that collect data on national notifiable diseases, vital statistics (birth or death certificates), and disease registries.

Types of Surveillance

Epidemiologists utilize different types of surveillance when searching for cases and identifying sudden outbreaks or epidemics. Types of surveillance include the following:

- **Active surveillance:** Involves having a research team go out into the community and look for cases of disease. It is very accurate but also expensive.
- **Passive surveillance**: Relies on existing reporting systems.
- **Digital surveillance**: Refers to Web crawling to identify reports of disease. This electronic monitoring is a relatively new method that looks online for reports of symptoms in multiple countries and languages. The **Global Public Health Intelligence Network** is an electronic public health early warning system developed by Canada's Public Health Agency and is part of the **World Health Organization's Global Outbreak Alert and Response Network.**
- **Sentinel surveillance**: Monitors a special community to look for changes in distribution of disease. Usually used when passive surveillance systems would not be effective and is conducted in a small location, such as an existing hospital, to identify new trends that warrant further study—for example, the **National Institute for Occupational Safety and Health's Sentinel Event Notification System for Occupational Risks (SENSOR).**

PRACTICE QUESTIONS

To test your knowledge of the tasks in this section, review the following questions.

1. The terms incidence and prevalence are used for different reasons. For example, if a hospital administrator needs to know how many beds should be available to treat specific disease states, this reflects the _____ . (Fill in the blank.)

Answer: Prevalence, because this includes all cases.

2. The same hospital administrator needs to know the postoperative infarction rate in the cardiothoracic surgery department during May 2017. What epidemiologic measure does the administrator need?

Answer: Incidence rate, because this includes new cases in a particular time period.

3. The prevalence of disease is correlated with the incidence and how long the person has the disease. The relationship is as follows: Prevalence = Incidence × Duration. How is the prevalence of disease impacted by the introduction of a new medication that improves survival?

    a. The prevalence goes up.
    b. The prevalence goes down.
    c. The prevalence stays the same.

Answer: a. The prevalence goes up. This is because more individuals will live.

4. A physician practicing in a US city begins to notice that people are coming to his office complaining of blurry vision. The physician looks back at his records and discovers that many of these patients were eventually diagnosed with diabetes. This physician conducted what kind of study?

Answer: Case series. These are reports of conditions, and there is no comparison group.

5. A group of factory workers were exposed to a toxic chemical. The employer is concerned that these workers may eventually develop lung disease (chronic obstructive pulmonary disease or asthma). What type of study design should the employer use to determine if the workers develop these lung diseases?

Answer: Cohort. This is a type of study in which the population is followed forward, the groups are assigned on the basis of exposure status, and exposure status was not assigned by the researcher, as in experimental studies. Assigning exposure status through an experimental study format would have been unethical.

6. A researcher wants to study risk factors for lung cancer in women. Lung cancer is a rare disease in women. The researcher matches lung cancer cases with women of the same age and race. The women matched with the lung cancer patients do not have lung cancer. Surveys are administered to both groups of women to determine their past exposures. What is this study design?

Answer: Case–control. The researcher is reviewing people with and without the disease. The study groups are determined by outcome status.

7. The World Health Organization is interested in folate consumption in developing countries. They want to examine the association between per-capita folate consumption and rates of colon cancer in each country. What is this study design?

Answer: Ecological. The data are being obtained at the aggregate and not the individual level.

Case study: *Maria Cordova is a 51-year-old woman living in El Paso, Texas. She emigrated from Mexico 10 years ago with her husband, Eduardo, and her two sons, Manuel and Ricardo. Recently, she has been very concerned because Eduardo has been complaining about blurred vision. He is also very thirsty all day. Although the Cordovas are undocumented residents of the United States, they were able to get an appointment at La Vida, a local health clinic that serves low-income residents. Veronica Rodriguez, the physician, examined Eduardo and performed a fasting glucose test, which had a result of 140 milligrams per deciliter. She explained to Maria that Eduardo has diabetes. This diagnosis was not uncommon; recent research has found the rates of diabetes to be higher among Mexican Americans than among non-Hispanic white Americans. (7.7% vs. 5.2%).*

Maria was very worried and asked Dr. Rodriguez what they could do as they did not have any health insurance. Dr. Rodriguez explained they have a community study (Project Risk) that is examining risk factors for diabetes in Mexican Americans. She also explained that if Eduardo enrolled in that study, they would be able to monitor his disease. He would also learn about diabetes, nutrition, and physical activity. Dr. Rodriguez provided the phone number for the study. Eduardo called the study office and found out he met the eligibility criteria and enrolled in the study. He remained in the study for one year.

The community research enrolled 240 people in the study: 120 individuals had newly diagnosed diabetes and 120 did not have diabetes. At the start of the study, researchers administered questionnaires, did physical examinations, and drew blood samples. One of the goals of the study was to examine the risk factors for diabetes between the two groups. They measured blood pressure, total cholesterol, low-density lipoprotein cholesterol, high-density lipoprotein cholesterol, hemoglobin A1c (HbA1c), physical activity, smoking habits, highest level of education completed (e.g., high school, bachelor's degree, graduate degree/professional degree), and income. HbA1c is the test used to test glucose levels over a two to three month period.[11]

Baseline characteristics of the population enrolled in this study are shown in the following table:

Baseline Characteristics of Participants in the Project Risk Study:

Characteristic	Newly Diagnosed Diabetes	No Diabetes
Age in years	60.5	55.7
% with hypertension	35	21
% with hyperlipidemia	40	14
HbA1c levels (%)	8.8	6.0
Mean number of minutes of activity per week	65	120
% smokers	15	7

Source: Based on Rodríguez-Saldaña.[11]
Note: HbA1c = hemoglobin A1c.

8. What is the study design for Project Risk?

Answer: Case–control study. Groups are assigned according to outcome status.

9. Will you report an OR or RR for data in this study?

Answer: OR. Case–control studies use ORs because you do not have incidence data. As you are selecting participants on the basis of outcome status, you are unable to calculate the "risk" of outcome attributable to exposure.

10. a. Set up a 2 × 2 table comparing smokers (n = 120) with nonsmokers (n = 120).

b. Of the 120 participants with diabetes, 15% are smokers. Of the 120 participants without diabetes, 7% are smokers.

c. Calculate the appropriate measure of association.

d. Interpret your findings

Answers:

	Diabetes	No Diabetes	Total
Smoking	18	8	26
No smoking	102	112	214
Total	120	120	240

$$OR = (18 \times 112) / (8 \times 102) = 2.47$$

People with diabetes are 2.47 times more likely to be smokers compared with people without diabetes.

B. Concepts of Biostatistics

INTRODUCTION

This section is Part B of the domain Evidence-Based Approaches to Public Health. In this section, we will focus on a more detailed discussion of biostatistical concepts that will be critical to your success as a public health professional. A detailed breakdown of statistical tests and their usage is found in Table 1-4.

Statistical principles are applied to a wide range of disciplines ranging from medicine to actuarial sciences. Although these disciplines are each quite divergent, they all depend on the field of applied mathematics for the processes of collecting information, analyzing data, drawing inferences, and reaching conclusions.[12] This is where statistics proves to be useful as it provides researchers with the tools to perform these functions. Biostatistics, or the field of statistics applied to medicine, public health, or biology, acts as a cornerstone for public health practice as it can be used in many capacities, including, but not limited to (1) assessing the effectiveness of an intervention, (2) identifying high-risk subpopulations during a disease outbreak, and (3) understanding the variation of a health indicator across a population.[12]

The field of biostatistics can be split into two realms that work concertedly: **descriptive statistics** and **inferential statistics.** Descriptive statistics, as the name implies, is the process of describing data. This involves taking raw data and providing summarizing information or depicting the data through various figures. Descriptive statistics is most often performed on a small subset of a **population**, known as a **sample**. Inferential statistics builds on descriptive statistics and allows researchers to draw conclusions on the

Table 1-4. Summary of Key Inferential Biostatistics Tests

Name of Test	Independent Variable	Dependent Variable	Tested Value	Null Hypothesis	Alternate Hypothesis	Other Considerations on When to Use
1-sample Z test	1 sample (comparing against a known value, a population parameter)	1 continuous variable	Mean	$H_0: \mu = \mu_1$	$H_A: \mu \neq \mu_1$ (2-sided) $H_A: \mu > \mu_1$ $H_A: \mu < \mu_1$ (1-sided)	The sample size needs to be greater than 30.
1-sample t test	1 sample (comparing against a known value, a population parameter)	1 continuous variable	Mean	$H_0: \mu = \mu_1$	$H_A: \mu \neq \mu_1$ (2-sided) $H_A: \mu > \mu_1$ $H_A: \mu < \mu_1$ (1-sided)	The sample size can be fewer than 30 observations.
1-sample Z test for dichotomous variable	1 sample (comparing against a known value, a population parameter)	1 dichotomous variable	Proportion	$H_0: p = p_0$	$H_A: p \neq p_0$ (2-sided) $H_A: p > p_0$ $H_A: p < p_0$ (1-sided)	The sample size needs to be greater than 10 for each of the categories of the dichotomous variable.
1-sample t test for dichotomous variable	1 sample (comparing against a known value, a population parameter)	1 dichotomous variable	Proportion	$H_0: p = p_0$	$H_A: p \neq p_0$ (2-sided) $H_A: p > p_0$ $H_A: p < p_0$ (1-sided)	The sample size can be fewer than 30 observations.

Table 1-4. (Continued)

Name of Test	Independent Variable	Dependent Variable	Tested Value	Null Hypothesis	Alternate Hypothesis	Other Considerations on When to Use
2-sample Z test	2 different groups (a dichotomous variable; e.g., men and women); 2 treatment groups (e.g., hypertension and normal blood pressure groups)	1 continuous variable	Means	$H_o: \mu_1 = \mu_2$	$H_A: \mu_1 \neq \mu_2$ (2-sided) $H_A: \mu_1 > \mu_2$ $H_A: \mu_1 < \mu_2$ (1-sided)	The sample size needs to be greater than 30 observations.
1-way ANOVA	3 or more different groups (if a nominal variable), or 3 or more different treatment or exposure levels (if an ordinal variable)	1 continuous variable	Means	$H_o:$ $\mu_1 = \mu_2 = \mu_3 \ldots$	$H_A: H_o$ is not true. $\mu_1 \neq \mu_2$ and/or $\mu_2 \neq \mu_3$ and/or $\mu_1 \neq \mu_3 \ldots$	The 1-way ANOVA will not tell you which of the alternate hypotheses you are rejecting the null hypotheses in favor of. Further analysis is necessary.
χ^2 test for goodness of fit	2 different groups (a dichotomous variable); 3 or more different groups (if a nominal variable); or 3 or more different treatment or exposure levels (if an ordinal variable)	1 categorical variable (nominal or ordinal)	Proportions or cell counts	The data are consistent with a specified or expected distribution.	The data are not consistent with a specified or expected distribution	When you have a known set of proportions with which to compare, such as racial makeup in a sample compared with census data.
χ^2 test for independence	1 categorical variable (nominal or ordinal)	1 categorical variable (nominal or ordinal)	Proportions or cell counts	In the sample, the 2 categorical variables are independent.	In the sample, the 2 categorical variables are not independent.	
Mann-Whitney U test	2 different groups (a dichotomous variable; e.g., men and women); 2 treatment groups (hypertension and normal blood pressure groups)	A continuous variable; data not normally distributed	U statistic (based on the ranks of the data points)	$H_o:$ the populations are equal.	$H_A:$ the populations are not equal.	

Table 1-4. (Continued)

Name of Test	Independent Variable	Dependent Variable	Tested Value	Null Hypothesis	Alternate Hypothesis	Other Considerations on When to Use
Sign test	2 different groups, but not independent groups	Continuous variable; data not normally distributed	Median difference	H_0: median difference is 0.	H_A: median difference is not 0.	It is insufficient for the 2 samples to be the same size. Each of the members of each group needs to be *dependent* on a member from the other group. This test is often used in tests comparing before-and-after readings on the same individual or some twin studies. Unlike the Wilcoxon signed-rank test, the Sign test only considers the direction of difference.
Wilcoxon signed-rank test	2 different groups, but not independent groups	Continuous variable; data not normally distributed	Median difference	H_0: median difference is 0.	H_A: median difference is not 0.	It is insufficient for the 2 samples to be the same size. Each of the members of each group needs to be *dependent* on a member from the other group. This test is often used in tests comparing before-and-after readings on the same individual or some twin studies. Unlike the Sign test, the Wilcoxon signed-rank test considers both the magnitude and the direction of difference.
Kruskal-Wallis test	3 or more different groups (if a nominal variable) or 3 or more different treatment or exposure levels (if an ordinal variable)	Continuous variable; data not normally distributed	H test statistic based on the median values between groups and rank	H_0: the 3 population medians are equal.	H_A: the 3 population medians are not equal.	

Table 1-4. (Continued)

Name of Test	Independent Variable	Dependent Variable	Tested Value	Null Hypothesis	Alternate Hypothesis	Other Considerations on When to Use
Simple linear regression models	1 variable (most often continuous, can be ordinal)	1 continuous variable	Mean, of dependent variable at levels of the independent variable	$H_0: \beta_1 = 0$	$H_1: \beta_1 \neq 0$	
Multiple linear regression models	2 or more variables (can be continuous, ordinal, or nominal if dummy variables are used)	1 continuous variable	Mean, of dependent variable at levels of the independent variables	$H_0: \beta_1 = 0$ and $\beta_2 = 0$ and $\beta_3 = 0 \ldots$	$H_0: \beta_1 \neq 0$ and $\beta_2 \neq 0$ and $\beta_3 \neq 0 \ldots$	
Logistic regression models	1 or more variables (can be continuous, ordinal, or nominal if dummy variables are used)	1 dichotomous variable	Log-odds ratio	$H_0: \beta_1 = 0$ and $\beta_2 = 0$ and $\beta_3 = 0 \ldots$	$H_0: \beta_1 \neq 0$ and $\beta_2 \neq 0$ and $\beta_3 \neq 0 \ldots$	
Survival analysis with survival curves	1 or more variables	Time-to-event data	S(t)	$H_0: S_1(t) = S_2(t)$ or the 2 survival curves are identical.	$H_1: S_1(t) = S_2(t)$ or the 2 survival curves are not identical.	
Log-rank test	1 or more variables	Time-to-event data	Log-rank test statistic (χ^2 distribution)	$H_0:$ relapse-free time is identical between the 2 groups.	$H_1:$ relapse-free time is not identical between the 2 groups.	

Note: ANOVA = analysis of variance.

population based on information collected from the sample. This section will help you sharpen the statistical skills needed to be certified in public health.

MAJOR CONTENT
Concepts of Descriptive Statistics
Characteristics of Variables

When researchers collect data for a study, they specify beforehand which characteristics of their subjects they are interested in for analysis. Biostatisticians refer to these characteristics as **variables**. For example, in a study in which researchers are trying to determine if a drug increases the risk for cardiovascular disease, they may focus on the specific variables of systolic and diastolic blood pressure. They may also collect information on other variables, such as gender, race, and age. They direct their attention toward these variables, and ignore other variables that may not be pertinent to their research, such as the make and model of the study participant's car.

A summarizing characteristic of a sample's variable is referred to as a **statistic**. This may be confusing as the term is also used for the field of study as a whole. Descriptive statistics is a key aspect of public health research, with the descriptive statistics of the study sample usually appearing at the beginning of a research publication. The field of inferential statistics utilizes the data from summarizing statistics to make inferences about those same characteristics at the level of the population, known as **parameters** (see Figure 1-5).

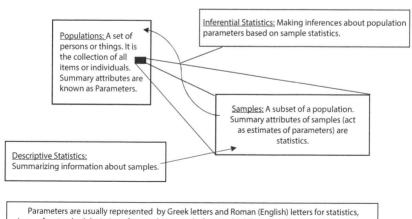

Figure 1-5. Relationship Between Inferential and Descriptive Statistics

Depending on the type of the variable, different analyses can be performed and different summarizing statistics can be obtained. The types of variables are characterized by the type of data that is collected and the scale of measurement that is used (see Figure 1-6):

1. **Nominal variables** (also known as **categorical variables**): Data are collected on the category in which the participant falls. The categories of the variable have no inherent order (e.g., race).

2. **Dichotomous variables**: Dichotomous variables are a specific type of variable that have only two possible values (e.g., exposure status as exposed or unexposed).

3. **Ordinal variables:** Similar to nominal variables, but the categories have an inherent order (e.g., socioeconomic level or level of education).

4. **Continuous variables:** Variables that can theoretically take any value between a minimum and maximum value.

   a. **Interval variables**: Interval variables are a type of continuous variable that have a distinct order and clearly defined intervals. They lack a *true zero*, or a zero value that is equivalent to an absence of the variable. The values also fail to reveal ratios of amounts (e.g., pH is an example of an interval variable, because a pH value of 0 does not mean absence of acidity, and a solution with a pH of 2 does not have twice the acidity of a solution with a pH of 1).

   b. **Ratio variables**: Ratio variables are similar to interval variables, but they have a true zero and values of the variable act as true ratios of one another (e.g., temperature in Kelvins).

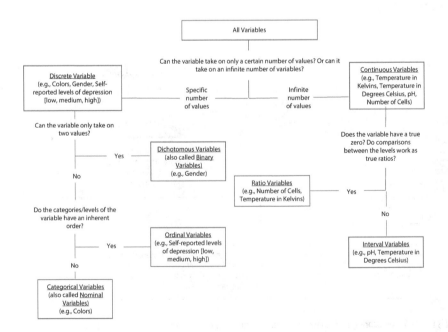

Figure 1-6. Types of Statistical Variables

Table 1-5. Commonly Used Descriptive Statistical Methods

Type of Variable	Nominal (Categorical)/ Dichotomous (Binary) Variables	Ordinal Variables	Continuous Variables
Summary statistics used	Frequency, relative frequency	Frequency, relative frequency, cumulative frequency, cumulative relative frequency	Mean, median, standard deviation, quartiles, range
Graphical types used to interpret	Bar chart, pie chart	Histogram	Box and whisker plots

It is important to note that a continuous variable can be collapsed into an ordinal or dichotomous variable for analysis. An example of this would be blood pressure readings that are characterized as hypotensive, normal, prehypertensive, type I hypertensive, or type II hypertensive (ordinal variable) or as normal or abnormal blood pressure readings (dichotomous variable). Collapsing variables can result in a loss of information but may be useful if you want to display the data in a specific format. Each type of variable has specific types of summary statistics that biostatisticians use with different types of graphical representations. The types of summarizing statistics and graphical methods used for each variable type are presented in Table 1-5.

Summary Statistics

Summary statistics are useful for displaying data in numerical or tabular format. The values are useful as they form the metric that is later applied to inferential statistics. Biostatisticians use specific types of summary statistics depending on the type of data collected:

1. **Frequency tables**: Frequency tables are used for nominal and ordinal variables. They reveal important information on the **frequency**, **relative frequency**, **cumulative frequency**, and **cumulative relative frequency** of the categories of the variables. Cumulative frequencies and cumulative relative frequencies are only relevant for ordinal variables (see Table 1-6).
2. **Measures of central tendency**: Continuous variables utilize measures of central tendency to give single values that describe the entire set of data. The commonly used measures of central tendency are the mean, median, and mode.
   a. **Mean**: The mean is the arithmetic average of the data set calculated as the sum of total values divided by the number of data values.
   b. **Median**: The median is the middle value of the data set when the data points are ordered by numerical value. If the data set has an even number of values, it is the arithmetic average of the two middle values of the data set.
   c. **Mode**: The mode is the most common value of the data set.
3. **Measures of variability**: While the measures of central tendency provide a single numerical value that is representative of the data set, it fails to show how much the

Table 1-6. Frequency Table for the Number of Chicken Pox Cases in an Elementary School

	Number of Cases of Chicken Pox per Grade			
	Frequency	Relative Frequency	Cumulative Frequency	Cumulative Relative Frequency
Kindergarten	22	0.407	22	0.407
1st grade	12	0.222	34	0.629
2nd grade	9	0.167	43	0.796
3rd grade	6	0.111	49	0.907
4th grade	3	0.056	52	0.963
5th grade	2	0.037	54	1
Total	54	1		

individual values of the data set deviate from this metric. Measures of variability provide information on the spread of the data set.

a. **Variance** (s^2) and **standard deviation** (s) are the most common measures used to inform on variability. Sample standard deviation can be calculated with the following formula. The variance is the value of the standard deviation squared.

$$s = \sqrt{\frac{1}{n-1} \sum_{i=1}^{n} (X_i - \bar{X})^2} \, ,$$

where $\{X_i, i = 1, 2, \ldots, n\}$ are the sample observations and $\bar{X}$ is the sample mean.

4. **Quartiles** and **range**: Quartiles and range are measures also used for continuous variables. **Quartiles** are the 25% and 75% values of the data set. The 25% value is calculated as the value in between the median and the lowest value when the data points are ordered in numerical value. The 75% value is calculated as the value in between the median and the highest value when the data points are ordered in numerical value. The spectrum of values in between the 25% value and the 75% value is termed the **interquartile range**. The interquartile range is also a useful value used to determine if there are any outliers in the dataset. The **range** is defined as the spectrum of values in between the lowest and highest values.

Displaying Data

The realm of descriptive statistics depends on displaying data and summarizing information in a meaningful way for audiences. Similar to the summary statistics used, the type of variable used assigns what type of graphical methods encapsulate the data set (see Figure 1-7):

- **Pie charts**: Pie charts are used for nominal variables. They display information on the relative frequency of each of the categories of the nominal variable.

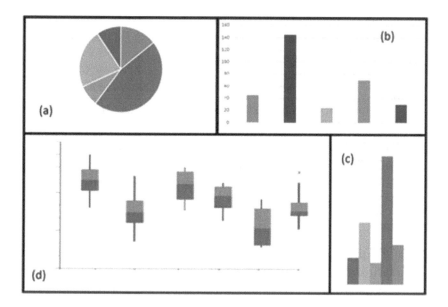

Figure 1-7. Visual Representations of Data: (a) Pie Charts, (b) Bar Graphs, (c) Histograms, and (d) Box and Whisker Plots

- **Bar charts**: Bar charts are used for nominal variables. They display information on the frequency of each of the categories of the nominal variable.
- **Histograms**: Histograms are used for ordinal variables. They also display information on the frequency of the categories of the ordinal variable. Unlike bar charts, however, the bars are placed adjacent to one another in the order of the ordinal variable's scale.
- **Box and whisker plots**: Box and whisker plots are useful for continuous variables. They provide information on the 25th and 75th percentile values of the data, the median, and the values of any outliers.

Concepts of Inferential Statistics

Probabilities

Probability is a central concept of inferential statistics. **Probability** is a numerical value applied to the likelihood for the occurrence of an event. All probabilities are proportions and therefore are calculated as a decimal value between the values of 0 and 1, or as a percentage between 0% and 100%:

$$P(\text{Characteristic}) = \frac{\text{\# of Individuals With Characteristic}}{\text{\# of Total Individuals in Sample/Population}}$$

Conditional probabilities build on this concept by assessing the probability of a characteristic given another characteristic. It considers the probability of the occurrence of an event in a subset of the entire population:

$$P(A|B) = \frac{\text{\# of Individuals With Characteristic A and B}}{\text{\# of Total Individuals in Sample/Population With Characteristic B}}$$

Examples of commonly used conditional probabilities in public health include the calculations of the **sensitivity, specificity, negative predictive value**, and **positive predictive values** of screening tests (see Section A of this chapter for more information on screening).

Independence

Closely related to the concept of probability is **independence**. Independence, as the term implies, is used to define a circumstance when the probability of one event does not have an impact on the probability of another event. Testing for the independence of two events is performed through assessing conditional probabilities: if A and B are independent,

$$P(A|B) = P(A)$$

and

$$P(B|A) = P(B)$$

Probability Models: Binomial Distribution and Normal Distribution

Probability models develop the concept of probability further and allow us to calculate the probability of outcomes by using mathematical formulas when it is impossible to calculate the exact probability because of the size of the sampling frame. Two common probability models that are used are the following:

1. **Binomial distribution**: A model of the distribution of a dichotomous outcome variable, such as testing positive or negative for a disease.
2. **Normal distribution** (also known as a **Gaussian distribution**): A model of the distribution of a continuous outcome variable, such as blood pressure.

The normal distribution is particularly important as it sets a series of assumptions about the data set that allow us to make inferences about a population from a sample and to test whether two samples are drawn from the same or different distributions. Comparing samples on the basis of these assumptions is a cornerstone of inferential biostatistics. Most of the tests that will be covered in this chapter depend on the underlying distribution being normal. Tests that depend on assumptions about the underlying distribution are known as **parametric tests**.

Assumptions of the Normal Distribution

There are several key characteristics of a normal distribution (see Figure 1-8):

- The mean, mode, and median are the same and are located at the center of the distribution.
- The distribution is symmetric around the median, mode, and mean. The distribution is therefore not **skewed**.
- The theoretical range extends horizontally from positive infinity to negative infinity.
- There are only two parameters necessary to describe a normal distribution: the mean and the standard deviation.
- The area under the curve of a normal distribution is exactly 1.0 or 100%. Approximately 68% of the area under the curve falls between −1 and +1 standard deviations from the mean, while approximately 95% of the curve falls between −2 and +2 standard deviations. Approximately 99% of the curve falls between −3 and +3 standard deviations.

Biostatisticians utilize a specific form of the normal distribution, known as the **standard normal distribution**, for calculations. This distribution has the parameters of a mean of 0.0 and a standard deviation of 1.0. Probabilities for the likelihood that a certain value or a more extreme value would be observed are tabulated through a **z scores table**, which is often used for inferential statistics analyses.

Other distributions that have been developed that fit data include the **Poisson distribution**, which is useful for count data. An example of count data is the number of hospitalizations among a certain group of patients. This distribution is right-skewed, because higher counts are less likely to be observed (i.e., most people will receive one or two hospitalizations). But someone in your sample might have had a serious illness and thus received 10 hospitalizations. Observed counts in a Poisson distribution tend to fall in the lower range of counts, with fewer observations in the higher range. Other nonnormal distributions are also often used in statistical analyses, such as the t, F, and χ^2 distributions.

Hypothesis Testing: Sampling Distributions

Inferential statistics depends on the concept of hypothesis testing. To perform hypothesis testing, one must understand how **sampling distributions** play a role. If you were to obtain the mean SAT score for a sample of 10 students from a high-school class in which the population mean aptitude test score was 1,000, you may get a wide range of values. The 10 sampled students might be the highest-scoring students and may have gotten an average of 1,600. Also, it is possible that the 10 sampled students may have been the lowest-scoring students, and may have gotten an average of around 400. However, if you continue to sample 10 random students from this same class of individuals, after performing 100 series of mean calculations from those various sets of 10 random students, you will begin to get a normal distribution of means, ranging from the minimum of 400

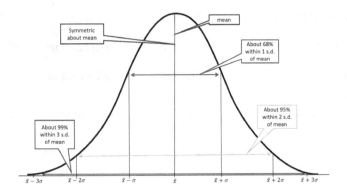

Note: s.d.=standard deviation.

Figure 1-8. Characteristics of a Normal Distribution

to a maximum of 1,600, but with a peak at around 1,000. Even if the raw data are not normally distributed, the **central limit theorem** states that, with repeated sampling, the individual mean calculations of samples form a normal distribution.

Hypothesis testing allows us to take a sample of another random 10 students from another high school, calculate their mean test score, and determine if the sample is statistically similar to the first high school with a mean test score of 1,000.

Hypothesis Testing: Null and Alternate Hypotheses

One of the key principles of inferential statistics is **hypothesis testing**. Hypothesis testing depends on testing two contrasting hypotheses:

1. The **null hypothesis**, notated often as H_0, is a precise statement.
2. The **alternate hypothesis** (also known as the **research hypothesis**) is a more ambiguous statement that rivals the null hypothesis.

Hypothesis Testing: Rejecting and Failing to Reject the Null Hypothesis

Similar to how our judicial system does not "prove innocence," hypothesis testing is based on the concept of finding enough evidence to reject the null hypothesis or, alternatively, failing to find enough evidence to reject the null hypothesis. In this manner, the field of biostatistics takes a conservative approach to analyzing the null hypothesis. Just as a defendant will be assessed as either "guilty" or "not guilty," the results of a biostatistical analysis culminate in the researcher "rejecting" or "failing to reject" the null hypothesis in favor of the alternate hypothesis.

P-values are probability values that measure the likelihood of obtaining the observed statistic or more extreme values when the null hypothesis is true. As deciding whether to reject or fail to reject the null hypothesis depends on this likelihood, researchers have to determine before performing their study what their benchmark for rejection needs to be. This is called the **level of significance** or **alpha (α)** value. Researchers often use the 0.05 level of significance for studies, but the more stringent 0.01 or the less stringent 0.10 are also used. Although the choice of setting the level of significance may vary, it is always assigned before performing the study.

Researchers also decide whether to perform a **one-sided test** or **two-sided test**. A one-sided test refers to the sample deviating from the null hypothesis conditions in one specific direction, such as being significantly greater than or significantly less than the null's means. The two-sided test does not specify directionality, and therefore is more conservative in its approach. This choice of directionality is also done before performing the study as the benchmark for rejecting or failing to reject the null hypothesis based on the p-value varies depending on whether a one-sided or two-sided test is performed.

After obtaining the results from the study, the researcher compares the p-value to the level of significance applied in the study. If the p-value is greater than alpha, the researcher fails to reject the null hypothesis. If the p-value is less than alpha, the researcher rejects the null hypothesis.

One-Sample Tests for the Means of a Continuous Response Variable

One-sample z tests are an important beginning point for hypothesis testing. This is a form of hypothesis testing that is performed on a continuous response variable. Consider the example of obtaining a sample of 50 adults with a mean systolic blood pressure of 155 millimeters of mercury (mm Hg). With information on the population's mean systolic blood pressure of 120 mm Hg and a standard deviation of 10 mm Hg, one can test whether the sample's systolic blood pressure was statistically different from the population's mean of 120 mm Hg. See the following formula for calculating the z score:

$$z = \frac{\overline{X} - \mu}{\sigma / \sqrt{n}}$$

Nonnormal Distributions: t Distributions

While z distributions are useful for when data on population means (μ) and standard deviations are available, this information is usually unavailable. This is when t distributions prove to be useful. There is an infinite number of t distributions that differ depending on the size of the obtained sample. The t distribution used depends on the **degrees of freedom**. For the one-sample t test, the degrees of freedom are $n - 1$, or the number of observations minus one. We can use the sample standard deviation as a substitution for the population's standard deviation. Although the standard deviation calculated from the sample (the statistic s) is different from the standard deviation from the population (the parameter σ), it acts as a useful substitute (see Figure 1-9).

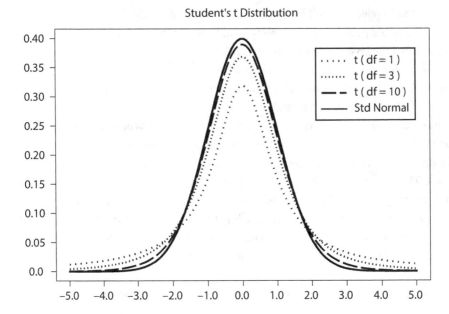

Figure 1-9. Different *t* Distributions Based on the Degrees of Freedom

When to Use a z Distribution or a t Distribution

If your sample is adequately large, the sample standard deviation (s) is a sufficient estimator of the population standard deviation (σ). "Adequately large" is a subjective term, but in general practice, statisticians will assume their sample is adequately large if they have at least 30 observations. In fact, the higher the value of n and thus the higher degrees of freedom, the closer a *t* distribution resembles a *z* distribution. At around an n of 30 (29 degrees of freedom), the *t* distribution is close enough to the *z* distribution that it makes no significant difference. In this case, the *z* test can be used, as your sample standard deviation should be close enough to the population standard deviation that your *z* statistic will follow a *z* distribution. If your sample has fewer than 30 observations and the population standard deviation is unknown, as is often the case, then a *t* test and a *t* distribution are the appropriate choices for your test of statistical inference.

Type I Errors, Type II Errors, Power

When one is performing hypothesis testing, two types of errors can occur. These include rejecting a true null hypothesis (**type I error**) or failing to reject a false null hypothesis (**type II error**; see Table 1-7).

As you can see from Figure 1-10,[13] where the biostatistician decides to determine the cutoff point for rejecting or failing to reject the null hypothesis will inversely impact the

Table 1-7. Type I and Type II Errors

Decisions of Hypothesis Testing	H₀ (Assumed Truth)	
	If the Null Is True	If the Null Is False
Reject the null	Type I error (α)	Power = $1-\beta$ (correct decision)
Fail to reject the null	$1-\alpha$ (correct decision)	Type II error (β)

ability to make a type I or a type II error. By shifting the cutoff to the right, the biostatistician decreases the likelihood of making a type I error but increases the likelihood of making a type II error, and vice versa.

Of the two types of errors, biostatisticians prefer type II to type I errors. Failing to reject a null hypothesis is a more conservative statement than rejecting the null hypothesis. It errs on the side of caution and can usually be rectified with further studies. Performing a type I error, however, involves incorrectly rejecting the null in favor of the alternate hypothesis. It falsely supports a novel research hypothesis or idea, which is far more problematic.

Power is an important concept that is related to type II errors. If β is the probability of falsely failing to reject the null hypothesis, then $1 - \beta$ is the probability of correctly rejecting the null hypothesis. This is the power of a study to correctly identify a deviation from the null hypothesis conditions. Power is dependent on several characteristics that can be manipulated to maximize the power of the study:

- **Increasing alpha (α)**: As stated previously, increasing the alpha will shift the cutoff for rejecting the null to the left. This will increase the power, but may also result in an increased likelihood for a type I error.
- **Increasing the effect size**: This deals with the effect of the conditions that cause a deviation from the conditions of the null (i.e., how far your sample mean is from the population mean). The researcher usually has no control over the effect of these conditions. In calculating power, a researcher typically will read through past studies or conduct a pilot study to get an estimate for how large of an effect size they can expect to observe in their study.
- **Increasing the sample size**: This is the method researchers usually use to obtain the power necessary for their study. Calculating the sample size necessary for a specific power therefore depends on the assigned (α), the desired power ($1 - \beta$), and the estimated effects size.

Confidence Intervals

Confidence intervals are closely related to the concept of hypothesis testing, and they form the second half of inferential statistics. Through hypothesis testing, one is able to use data from a sample to test whether the parameter for the population differs

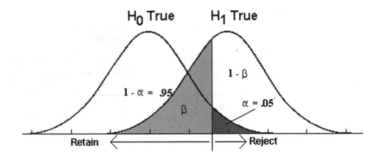

Source: Missouri State University.[13] Adapted with permission.
Figure 1-10. Distributions for Type I and Type II Errors

significantly from a value under the null hypothesis. Confidence intervals, however, use data from a sample to set upper and lower bounds to the estimate of a parameter.

Confidence intervals are often displayed using one of two formats:

1. (Lower limit, upper limit) or
2. Point estimate ± margin of error

In the second method of displaying the confidence interval, the two portions of the display consist of the **point estimate** and the **margin of error**. The point estimate, or the estimate of the population parameter, is the metric calculated from the sample. However, as this can deviate from the actual population parameter, the margin of error has a range in which one can estimate the actual parameter. There are two components to the margin-of-error calculation for the mean of a continuous variable:

1. The z score (or t score) corresponding to the area of the distribution that would match with the confidence interval
2. The standard error (SE) of the point estimate

The z score, the standard error, and the point estimate of the parameter all combined together form the confidence interval. The confidence interval can be displayed in the following format:

$$\text{Point Estimate} \pm z\, SE\, (\text{Point Estimate})$$

To understand what the confidence interval describes, think back to the basics of probabilities and the central limit theorem. Normal distributions reveal the likely distribution of sample means when one takes repeated measurements of random samples from a population. A 100% confidence interval of those sample means would range theoretically from $-\infty$ to $+\infty$. However, this information has no practical use for statistical purposes. Therefore, a 99%, 95%, or 90% confidence interval is far more useful for estimating the population parameter. Confidence intervals, therefore, build on our understanding of probabilities. A 95% confidence interval for a parameter means the following:

$$P \text{ (Lower Limit of Confidence Interval} < \text{Population Parameter}$$
$$< \text{Upper Limit of Confidence Interval)} = 0.95$$

Because estimation with confidence intervals and hypothesis testing go hand in hand, one is able to obtain the same results using either method. For example, if a parameter value under the null hypothesis falls outside of an obtained 95% confidence interval, one would reject the null hypothesis at the significance level of 0.05.

Confidence intervals are also used in the field of epidemiology to determine if there is a significant correlation between an exposure and an outcome. Epidemiologists do this by assessing if the value of 1.0 falls outside of the confidence interval range for an OR or an RR. This is because an OR or RR of 1.0 is the null value or the value you would observe under the null hypothesis that there is no difference in odds or risk. If 1.0 falls outside of the confidence interval, there is statistical significance for an increase or decrease in risk or odds. Confidence intervals can also show the strength of association between the exposure and the outcome (see Section A of this chapter for more information on RRs and ORs).

One-Sample Test for the Proportion of a Dichotomous Response Variable

One-sample z and t tests also can be performed for the proportion of a dichotomous variable. To perform this test, you will need at least 10 observations in each of the categories of the dichotomous variable. The proportion of occurrences of an event is usually calculated from x, the number of events, and n, the sample size:

$$\hat{p} = \frac{x}{n}$$

For testing the null hypothesis that $\hat{p} = p_0$, one can obtain the test statistic by using this formula:

$$z = \frac{\hat{p} - p_0}{\sqrt{p_0(1 - p_0)/n}}$$

Two-Sample Tests for the Means of a Continuous Response Variable

The previously mentioned parametric tests involve comparing a sample against a population. However, in much of public health research, the focus is often on comparing two samples. Perhaps you are comparing data from a control or placebo group against a group receiving a medication or comparing data from two cohorts of individuals who have or have not experienced an exposure. In these scenarios, the researcher is not trying to determine if the data correspond to a specific population, but whether the two data collections have been drawn from two statistically distinct populations. Therefore, your analysis when comparing two samples with a continuous response variable will be on whether there is a statistically significant difference between the means of the two samples, or in other words:

$$H_0: \mu_1 \neq \mu_2,$$

or, identically,

$$H_0: \mu_1 - \mu_2 = 0$$

The test statistic is therefore calculated similarly to the one-sample z and t tests. The numerator will be the difference of the two means. However, a complexity with the calculation of the test statistic for these two-sample tests is the denominator: what value would be appropriate for the sample size and for the standard deviation? The equations are complex and, therefore, most contemporary biostatisticians utilize software packages such as SAS and SPSS to perform these tests instead of calculating them by hand.

Similar to how one chooses to perform a z test or t test on the basis of sample size, one can use a z statistic score if both of the sample sizes are individually greater than or equal to 30. If even one sample size is less than 30, one can utilize a t statistic by using a degrees of freedom value of $n_1 + n_2 - 2$.

Matched-Pair Test

Examples of matched-pair analyses are *twin studies*, in which there is a twin in each sample group and measurements are made by comparing the two twins. Also, *before-and-after* clinical studies, in which individuals act as their own controls, are examples of studies in which a matched-pair test analysis can be performed. Readings are taken before an intervention and then after the intervention. The reason for using a matched-pair test in these scenarios is that the individual readings are not independent. Readings between twins and readings taken from the same individual at different points of time are related to one another.

In both of these scenarios, calculations are made *between* the pairs of readings. Therefore, the matched-pair test works like a one-sample test, with the data being the difference in readings between the pairs. For example, if before-and-after readings are taken from a blood pressure study in which readings were taken before treatment and after treatment, the value that would be analyzed for statistical significance is the difference in blood pressure readings.

Parametric Tests Comparing Two Proportions of a Dichotomous Response Variable

Similar to how we built on our understanding of one-sample tests with a continuous variable to two-sample tests with a continuous variable, we can also build on our previous knowledge to make comparisons about a dichotomous outcome variable between two samples. This has much clinical relevance, as many clinical outcome variables are dichotomous, such as if our patients are "alive" or "deceased." This can prove to be helpful if we are comparing a clinical sample group that is receiving a new treatment to another group that is receiving the standard treatment. How would we compare whether the proportions that are alive at 12 months are the same between the two groups? We would have to use a two-sample z test or two-sample t test for proportions.

Parametric Tests Comparing Three or More Means of a Continuous Response Variable

Analysis of variance (ANOVA) tests are conducted to compare means of three or more continuous variables by comparing the variation in the values of the members *within* each of the subsamples or groups drawn from the populations with the variance *between* the means of the groups. These two values are defined as the **sum of squares between (SSB)**, which is the sum of the squared differences of the means of each sample and the overall mean, and the **sum of squares error (SSE)**, which is the sum of the squared difference of each member of each sample with the sample mean. The sum of squares error is also sometimes referred **to sum of squares within (SSW)**. The **sum of squares total (SST)** reveals the difference in values of all the points from the total mean.[12]

The degrees of freedom of SSB is calculated as $df_1 = k - 1$, or the number of groups minus 1. The degrees of freedom of SSE is calculated as $df_2 = N - k$, or the number of data points minus the number of groups. These two values of SSB and SSE are standardized by dividing by their corresponding degrees of freedom to obtain the **mean squares between (MSB)** and the **mean squares error (MSE)**. The ratio of these two values provides the test statistic known as an **F statistic**. F statistics are analyzed for significance along an **F distribution**, which is a right-skewed distribution.[12]

An important note is that an ANOVA test cannot identify the specific mean that is significantly different from another. The null hypothesis is that

$$H_0: \mu_1 = \mu_2 = \mu_3 = \mu_4 \ldots$$

The tested alternate hypothesis is that H_0 is false. This may mean that $\mu_1 \neq \mu_2$, and/or $\mu_1 \neq \mu_3$, and/or $\mu_2 \neq \mu_3$. To determine the specific discordant pairs, two independent

Table 1-8. ANOVA Table

Source of Variation	Sum of Squares	Degrees of Freedom	Mean Squares	F Statistic
Between treatments	SSB	k – 1	MSB = SSB/k – 1	F = MSB/MSE
Error residual	SSE	N – k	MSE = SSE/N – k	
Total	SST = SSB + SSE	N – 1		

Note: ANOVA = analysis of variance; k = number of samples; MSB = mean squares between; MSE = mean squares error; N = total sample size; SSB = sum of squares between; SSE = sum of squares error; SST = sum of squares total.

samples tests could be further performed with the caution that multiple comparisons may result in an increased likelihood to perform a type I error.

The information from ANOVA tests is usually summated in an ANOVA table (see Table 1-8).

Chi-Squared (χ^2) Goodness-of-Fit

The **chi-squared (χ^2) goodness-of-fit** test is performed when one is comparing the proportions of a categorical variable against specified proportions. Consider a situation in which a professor teaches a class in which the distribution of grades is typically 25% As, 40% Bs, 15% Cs, and 20% Ds or lower. They can assess whether the distribution of grades for the current class fits the typical grade distribution. This test measures the difference between the observed proportions (O) and the expected proportions (E) based on the null hypothesis. For the test to be accurate, each of the categories has to have a count value greater than or equal to 5.

Once the test statistic is obtained, the χ^2 test statistic is assessed for significance on the χ^2 distribution table with degrees of freedom of k – 1, or the number of categories minus 1:

$$\chi^2 = \sum \frac{(O - E)^2}{E}, df = k - 1$$

$$E = P_{expected} * n$$

Tests Comparing the Proportions of Two Categorical Variables

The knowledge from a χ^2 goodness-of-fit test can be extended to comparing the proportions of two or more samples. The question that is being asked when one is dealing with two categorical variables is whether the two variables are independent or if they are associated or correlated. This is known as the **chi-square (χ^2) test of independence.**

From our understanding of proportions, independence can be tested by seeing if $P(A|B) = P(A)$ and $p(A|B) = P(A)$. To perform this test, we will need to calculate the **marginal frequencies.** The marginal frequencies reveal the frequency of that specific variable in the sample population (see Table 1-9).

Table 1-9. ANOVA Table

	Males	Females	Marginal Frequency
Pass	0.42	0.28	0.7
Fail	0.18	0.12	0.3
Marginal frequency	0.6	0.4	1.0

Note: ANOVA = analysis of variance.

If two variables are independent, then the cell counts will closely match the product of the marginal frequencies. Building on the example in which a professor wants to examine the distribution of grades in her class, the proportion of male students who have passing grades is $P_{Males\ \&\ Pass} = P_{Males} * P_{Pass}$.

This product of the marginal frequencies provides us with the expected count necessary for calculating the χ^2 test statistic. The χ^2 test is performed by assessing how different the overall expected cell and observed frequencies are from each other. The degrees of freedom equals $(r - 1)(c - 1)$, or the number of categories in the first variable minus 1 times the number of categories in the second variable minus 1.

Nonparametric Tests

Nonparametric tests, also known as distribution-free tests, require fewer assumptions about the underlying distribution of the population. They tend to be less powerful, but can be useful for heavily skewed data, such as small data sets with several prominent outliers. Examples of commonly used nonparametric tests are the following:

- **Mann-Whitney U test**: This test is performed on continuous outcome variables from two samples. It compares the ranks instead of the raw values of data between two samples. It is the nonparametric counterpart to the t and z tests.
- **Sign test:** This test is performed on continuous outcome variables from matched-pair samples. It is a nonparametric test that compares the direction of change between the two paired groups. It is the nonparametric counterpart to the matched-pair t and matched-pair z tests.
- **Wilcoxon signed-rank test:** This test is performed on continuous outcome variables from matched-pair samples. It is a nonparametric test that compares the magnitude and direction of change between the two paired groups. The addition of magnitude is the significant difference between the sign test and the Wilcoxon signed-rank test. It is also a nonparametric counterpart to the matched-pair t and matched-pair z test.
- **Kruskal-Wallis test:** This test is performed on continuous outcome variables from three or more samples. It compares the medians among the different samples. The Kruskal-Wallis test is the nonparametric counterpart to the one-way ANOVA test.

Multivariable Methods and Regression Analysis

So far, we have discussed ways of testing hypotheses on data for which the predictor (e.g., exposed status, gender) is categorical. In these tests the outcome has been categorical (e.g., disease status, letter grade in a class) or continuous (e.g., blood pressure, body mass index). But how does one test hypotheses on data when the predictor and the outcome are both continuous? This is where **linear regression** is necessary. In linear regression, the predictor is often called the **independent variable**, and the outcome is often called the **dependent variable**.

Simple Linear Regression

For simple linear regression to be performed, four assumptions have to be met:

1. **Linearity**: The relationship between the variables x and y is linear.
2. **Independence**: Each data observation is independent.
3. **Normality:** The residuals from each value of x are normally distributed.
4. **Heteroscedasticity:** There is constant variance of the errors at different values of x.

To understand how simple linear regression analysis works, the data can be presented graphically. The data can be placed on a plot so the independent variable is plotted along the x-axis and the dependent variable is plotted along the y-axis. Regression analysis involves calculating a linear line that describes the data using the least squares estimate method.

Residuals

No line that is produced for a linear regression will perfectly fit the data. There will be observations that fall above and below the line. The goal of a regression is to find the line that minimizes the distance between each observation and this line. The vertical distance between an observation and the line is called a **residual** or **residual error**. The plotted line that minimizes the sum of all the residuals is the best descriptor of the trend between your independent variable (x) and your dependent variable (y). Residuals can be thought of as a similar concept to variance. Variance describes the difference between individual observations and the mean. If the regression line is interpreted as the mean of the independent variable that changes with the value of your independent variable, then residuals are basically the variance between each observation and the mean at that value of x.

The **least squares estimate method** is the preferred method of finding the linear line that minimizes the **residuals** from each data point and the line along the y-axis. This method of calculating the regression line is usually not performed by biostatisticians by hand, and most often is completed with statistical software packages such as SAS and SPSS.

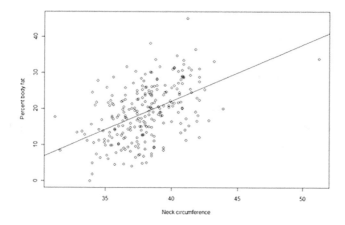

Source: Boston University.[14] Reprinted with permission.
Figure 1-11. Linear Regression of Data Comparing Neck Circumferences With Percentage Body Fat

The line is usually displayed in the following format:

$$y = mx + b$$

In this format, the value of the independent variable can be used to predict the value of the dependent variable. The two components necessary to predict y from x are the **intercept** (b) and the **slope** (m). The intercept, typically referred to in statistical applications as β_0 or b_0, is simply the predicted value of the dependent variable when the independent variable is valued at 0. The slope value, referred to in statistical applications as β_1 or b_1, is an important part of regression analysis in that it predicts the effect of the independent variable. A positive m value means that increases to the independent variable result in increases to the dependent variable, while a negative m value means that increases to the independent variable result in decreases to the dependent variable. For example, in Figure 1-11, if we obtain a slope value of +3.40, we can state that for every unit increase in neck circumference, there are 3.40 unit increases in percentage of body fat.[14]

The equation, however, does not describe the fit of the data. Two metrics that are used to measure the fit of the data are the following:

1. **Pearson product moment correlation coefficient** (*r*): This coefficient ranges from −1.0 to +1.0. It reveals both the fit of the data to the regression line and the direction of association between the variables. A negative *r* value states that as the values of the independent variable increase, the values of the dependent variable decrease. A positive value states that as the values of the independent variable increase, the values of the dependent variable also increase. The distance of the *r* value from 0 reveals the strength of the relationship. For example, a value of +0.9 or −0.9 both reveal a strong

positive and negative linear relationship between the variables, respectively. A value of +0.1 or –0.1 reveals a weak positive and negative linear relationship between the variables, respectively.

2. **Coefficient of determination (r^2):** For simple linear regressions, this is the squared value of the Pearson product moment correlations coefficient. It standardizes the value to be used as a metric of the fit of the linear regression model for both positively and negatively associated variables. This value is often obtained through the use of statistical software. The range of values for the coefficient of determination is 0 to 1.0.

Consider Figure 1-12, which depicts strong and weak linear associations of data. The Pearson product moment correlation coefficients for data sets 1 and 2 would both be positive, as there is a positive linear relationship between the independent and dependent variables for both data sets. However, the relationship demonstrated by 1 is stronger, meaning that the coefficient for data set 1 would be closer to 1.0 than the coefficient for data set 2. The coefficient for data set 4, on the other hand, would be negative, because of the inverse relationship between the independent and dependent variable. A linear regression analysis for the data from scatter plot 3 would have a value close to 0 because of the poor linear relationship between the variables.

Often biostatisticians are not simply interested in analyzing the effect of one predictor variable from a study. Even in clinical trials that study the impact of just one drug, researchers may be interested in the impact of confounding characteristics or the effect modification of another variable. We can extend the principles from simple linear regression analysis to perform **multiple linear regression analysis**.

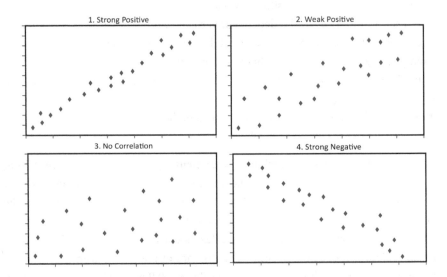

Figure 1-12. Strong and Weak Linear Associations of Data

Unlike simple linear regression analysis, it is difficult to graphically display the equation obtained from a multiple linear regression analysis. The equation, however, can be written in the following format:

$$y = b_0 + b_1 x_1 + b_2 x_2 + b_3 x_3 \ldots$$

The b_0 value, similar to in the simple linear regression model, is the intercept, or the value of the dependent variable when all of the independent variables equal 0. The individual slope statistics ($b_1, b_2, b_3, \ldots$) reveal the impact of each individual independent variable on the dependent variable. Statistical analyses can be performed to reveal the significance of each independent variable. Such analyses allow for the test of the impact of confounders (usually displayed as individual $b_n x_n$ variables) or effect modifiers (usually displayed in a polynomial $b_n x_n x_{n+1}$ format).

Regression analyses also can be performed on dichotomous outcome variables. As dichotomous outcome variables can only have two values, the analysis is performed on the log OR of the probabilities of the dichotomous variable. This is known as **logistic regression analysis:**

$$\ln\left(\frac{\hat{p}}{1-\hat{p}}\right) = b_0 + b_1 x_1 + b_2 x_2 + b_3 x_3 \cdots$$

The logistic transformation allows a linear regression between the two sides of the equation. The interpretation of the b values is a little more complex though with logistic regression analysis. The b value predicts the expected change in the log odds relative to a one-unit change in x.

Survival Analysis

A very relevant field to clinical studies is **survival analysis**. Survival analysis works with a dichotomous outcome variable, such as mortality, but considers the effect over a continuous variable of time. This type of outcome variable is known as a **time-to-event variable.**

Consider a drug trial performed on cancer patients in which a new treatment A is compared against a currently available treatment B, as shown in Figure 1-13. At 21 weeks after treatment, there is a significant difference in mortality, but this diminishes by week 42. Survival analysis through time-to-event data considers survivorship at all points in time in a composite manner.

Time-to-event data have key characteristics:

- **Time-to-event data are always positive:** Negative or 0 values that reveal events that have occurred before or at the time of initiating the study are not included. The time to event is known as the **survival time.**
- **Censoring can occur:** Censoring occurs when participants drop out of the study, the study ends, or the participants are removed from the study population because of a competing outcome. We know the survival time is greater than the observed time, but

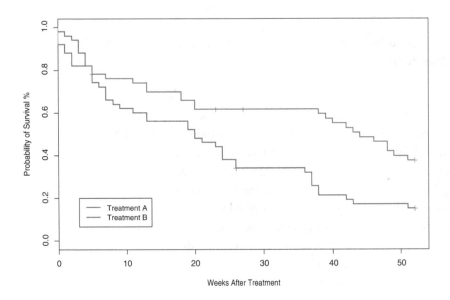

Figure 1-13. Survival Analysis of Treatment A and Treatment B

we do not know the true extent of the survival time. Data are included in the study up to the time of censoring. This length of time is known as **follow-up time**.

Kaplan-Meier curves provide a graphical display of survival data with study time on the x-axis and probability of surviving on the y-axis. Survivorship at each point of time is the probability that an individual will survive to the next time point, given that they have already survived up until now. It is thus calculated as a product of the probability of surviving at every time point before. As is shown in Figure 1-14, at each event, there are drops in survivorship, as would be expected.[15] This graph also shows censoring at time points through vertical dashes. As censoring does not have an impact on survivorship (as time-to-event information is unavailable for censored individuals), it does not result in dips in the line.

The **log-rank test** is a statistical analysis methodology that allows us to compare survivorship between two groups. It uses the same fundamental principles that we used for comparing independence between two categorical variables. The results of a log-rank test tell us whether survival curves differ over the course of the study and, thus, whether the probabilities of having an event at each time point differ between groups.

Using Statistical Packages or Software to Analyze Data

Although it is still possible to analyze data manually, one often needs to use software packages for sophisticated statistical analyses. In addition, statistical software packages make data storage and organization and transfer much easier.

Public health research and application are highly interdisciplinary and employ a variety of quantitative and qualitative methods. There are many statistical software packages

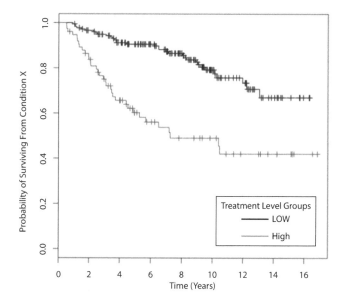

Source: Loi et al.[15] The figure was adapted from the original, available at: https://doi.org/10.1186/1471-2164-9-239, an open access article distributed under the terms of the Creative Commons Attribution License.

Figure 1-14. Kaplan-Meier Curve

available. Some are designed for general analytic methods and the others could be more specialized. It is not easy to pick the right one to use. Recent studies revealed that SAS, Stata, and SPSS are three leading software packages used in quantitative health research and Nvivo, Atlas ti, and QDA are top qualitative analysis packages.[16]

PRACTICE QUESTIONS

To test your knowledge of the tasks in this section, review the following case study and questions.

Case study: *Jackie is performing a study on children and teenagers who live in her apartment complex to obtain data on influenza vaccination history and other demographic information. She summarized the data of her findings in a table:*

Variable	Vaccinated (n = 713)	Unvaccinated (n = 809)
Mean age (no. of years ± margin of error)[a]	15.5 ± 0.7	13.7 ± 0.6
Male, %	49.1	52
College track, %	80.1	82.3
Mean no. of sick days since previous August (no. of days ± margin of error)[a]	4.2 ± 2.1	6.9 ± 3.1

[a]Margin of error was obtained for the 95% confidence interval.

1. Age would be considered what type of variable?
   a. Continuous
   b. Dichotomous
   c. Ordinal
   d. Nominal

Answer: a. Continuous. The variable can take any value in between a theoretical minimum and maximum.

2. What would be an example of an *ordinal* variable on which Jackie could have obtained information?
   a. Right-handed or left-handed
   b. Type of after-school activity in which the student participated
   c. Elementary-school age, middle-school age, freshman, sophomore, junior, or senior
   d. Number of minutes of commute each morning to school

Answer: c. Elementary-school age, middle-school age, freshman, sophomore, junior, or senior. These are well-defined categories that can be ranked in ascending or descending order.

3. If Jackie had 713 individuals in both groups, could she use a matched-pair *t* test with the above data to determine differences in mean ages between the two groups?
   a. Yes
   b. No

Answer: b. No. To perform a matched-pair *t* test, the values need to be associated in a specific manner that makes the readings not independent. This test is used either for twin studies or in before-and-after readings in epidemiologic studies of the same individuals.

4. Jackie calculates the point estimate and margin of error of the mean age of the vaccinated group as 15.5 ±0.7. What would be the center value of the 90% confidence interval?
   a. 14.4
   b. 20.1
   c. 15.5
   d. Cannot be determined from the given information

Answer: c. 15.5. The change in the confidence interval would only affect the margin of error, not the point estimate.

5. Would the 99% confidence interval be wider than, the same as, or narrower than the 95% confidence interval?
   a. Wider than the 95% confidence interval
   b. The same as the 95% confidence interval

c. Narrower than the 95% confidence interval

d. Cannot be determined from the given information

Answer: a. The range of possible values increases with the increase of the confidence level. Remember that a 100% confidence interval includes all values from a theoretical minimum and maximum. As your confidence interval level increases, it approaches this!

6. What would be the best method of visualizing the number of sick days in each group?

a. Box and whisker plot

b. Pie chart

c. Histogram

d. Bar chart

Answer: a. Box and whisker plots are most appropriate for continuous variables such as the number of sick days in each group.

7. The mean age of the vaccinated group is 15.5 years, but the median age is 13.9 years. From this information, we can assume what about the distribution for this variable?

a. It is most likely left-skewed

b. It is most likely right-skewed

c. It is most likely close to normally distributed.

d. We cannot make any assumptions about the distribution from the given information.

Answer: b. It is most likely right-skewed because of outliers at the higher end of the values, which would result in a lower median. The mean, which is more affected by outliers, would be skewed greater than the median.

8. If Jackie collected data also on the household income to determine if there was a significant difference between the vaccinated and unvaccinated groups and performed a test with income as the dependent variable, what would her null hypothesis be?

a. H_0: μ(income vaccinated) = μ(income unvaccinated)

b. H_0: μ(income vaccinated) ≤ μ(income unvaccinated)

c. H_0: μ(income vaccinated) ≥ μ(income unvaccinated)

d. H_0: μ(income vaccinated) ≠ μ(income unvaccinated)

Answer: a. The null hypothesis is a precise statement that states there is no statistical difference between samples or test groups.

9. If Jackie also obtained data on the number of doctor's visits in the past year between the vaccinated and unvaccinated groups and obtained a p-value of 0.035, and tested it against an $\alpha = 0.05$, she would:

a. Fail to reject the null hypothesis

b. Fail to reject the alternate hypothesis

c. Reject the null hypothesis

d. Reject the alternate hypothesis

Answer: c. Reject the null hypothesis. The p-value revealed that there was a statistical difference at an alpha $= 0.05$ level.

10. If Jackie wanted to test whether there was a statistically significant difference in the number of sick days between vaccinated and unvaccinated individuals, what test should she use?

a. χ^2 test of independence

b. χ^2 goodness-of-fit test

c. One-sample t test

d. Two-sample t test

Answer: d. Two-sample t test. The response variable is a continuous variable and there are two groups being compared with each other.

Jackie also collected information on how many siblings each person she interviewed had and placed the data in a probability table:

Name of Test	Independent Variable P(Vaccinated)	Dependent Variable P(Unvaccinated)
P(with 2 siblings)	a	b
P(with 3+ siblings)	c	d

11. Which one of the following would be an example of a statement that could be tested to determine if vaccination rates and number of siblings were independent?

a. P(vaccinated) × P(only child) = a

b. P(unvaccinated × P(with 1 sibling) = d

c. P(unvaccinated) = a

d. P(vaccinated) = P(unvaccinated)

Answer: a. P(vaccinated) × P(only child) = a. Independence usually can be determined through multiplication of marginal percentiles.

12. What is the range of r^2 values, coefficient of determination?

a. −1.0 to 1.0

b. 0 to 1.0

c. 1.0 to $+\infty$

d. $-\infty$ to $+\infty$

Answer: b. 0 to 1.0. r^2 values describe the fit of regression lines to data. A strong fit is closer to 1.0 and a weak fit is closer 0.0.

13. Jackie wants to perform a regression analysis to determine how a variety of predictor variables (e.g., age, gender, number of siblings) affect the *probability of being vaccinated or unvaccinated*. What type of regression analysis should she perform?

    a. Multiple linear regression analysis

    b. Survival analysis

    c. Multiple logistic regression analysis

    d. Regression analysis is not possible with multiple predictor variables

Answer: c. Multiple logistic regression analysis. The outcome variable is a dichotomous variable of being vaccinated or unvaccinated.

Jackie performs linear regression analysis to get the following formula: Y(number of days sick) $= \beta_1 X$*(number of siblings)* $+ \beta_0$*, where* $\beta_1 = 5.6$ *and* $\beta_0 = 2.1$.

14. What is the best interpretation of the β_1 value?

    a. For every increase of 1 unit of number of siblings, there is an increase of 5.6 sick days on average.

    b. For every increase of 1 unit of number of siblings, there is a decrease of 5.6 sick days on average.

    c. For every increase of 1 sick day, there is a decrease of 5.6 units of number of siblings on average.

    d. For every increase of 1 sick day, there is an increase of 5.6 units of number of siblings on average.

Answer: a. For every increase of 1 unit of number of siblings, there is an increase of 5.6 sick days on average. The β value is the slope, which refers to the number of units increase of *y* per 1 unit increase in *x*.

15. From the obtained regression analysis, what would Jackie assume is the average number of sick days in her study sample for individuals who had 0 siblings?

    a. 0.0

    b. 2.1

    c. 5.6

    d. 7.7

Answer: b. When there are 0 siblings, the *x* value equals 0, and therefore the *y* value will equal the intercept or β_0 value.

16. Jackie looks back to other statistical tests she has performed in the past year. She sees a one-way ANOVA test that she performed on the mean servings of veggies students ate, with samples from elementary school, middle school, and high school. If she had three sample groups, consisting of 32 elementary students, 20 middle-school students, and 15

high-school students, what are the degrees of freedom for the numerator and denominator of her one-way ANOVA table?

Answer: Numerator is k − 1, which is 3 − 1 = 2. The denominator degrees of freedom are N − k, or 67 − 3, or 64.

17. Another test Jackie performed last year was a chi-square test of independence, where she compared gender, recorded as male or female, against color of backpack, recorded as red, blue, white, black, yellow, or other. How many degrees of freedom were in her chi-square test of independence?

Answer: 5 degrees of freedom: $(r − 1)(c − 1) = (2 − 1)(6 − 1) = 5$.

18. Finally, Jackie performed a two-sample t test comparing the geography test scores between the boys and girls in her class. There were 22 boys and 19 girls. What were the degrees of freedom of her two-sample t test?

Answer: 39: $N_1 + N_2 − 2 = 22 + 19 − 2$.

CONCLUSION

In this chapter, several concepts and methods for evidence-based public health were reviewed. Appreciating how the evidence is generated, evaluated, and ultimately applied is essential for implementing public health interventions. The concepts reviewed in Section A of this chapter are the foundation of epidemiologic methods. Measures of disease frequency and association assess the scope of the public health problem. Evaluating sources of error in these measures allows us to assess the validity and reliability of the conclusions. Understanding diagnostic testing and screening provides the foundation for initiating or evaluating screening programs.

Biostatistics, or the field of statistics used to analyze data related to public health, medicine, and health care, is a crucial cornerstone to the practice of public health. The two realms of biostatistics—descriptive statistics and inferential statistics—work concertedly to analyze data from samples and to draw conclusions about the population from which the sample is drawn. Data for public health are coded in specific types of variables: nominal, ordinal, dichotomous, continuous, interval, and ratio. Depending on the type of variable, different statistical analyses can be performed. Decisions to use the proper test are necessary for the practice of public health. There are various types of tests that can be used to analyze the data collected from these data types including z tests, t tests, one-way ANOVA, and regression analysis. Understanding which tests are appropriate for the type of data that are collected is a key component of public health. The quantitative fields of epidemiology and biostatistics provide the methods necessary to evaluate the efficacy and effectiveness of many types of public health interventions.

REFERENCES

1. Brownson RC, Fielding JE, Maylahn CM. Evidence-based public health: a fundamental concept for public health practice. *Annu Rev Public Health*. 2009;30(1):175–201.

2. Partners in Information Access for the Public Health Workforce. Steps in searching and evaluating the literature. Available at: https://phpartners.org/tutorial/04-ebph/2-keyConcepts/4.2.5.html. Accessed December 16, 2017.

3. Centers for Disease Control and Prevention. Principles of epidemiology in public health practice, third edition: An introduction to applied epidemiology and biostatistics. 2012. Available at: https://www.cdc.gov/ophss/csels/dsepd/ss1978/lesson3/section1.html. Accessed April 20, 2018.

4. Aschengrau A, Seage GR. *Essentials of Epidemiology in Public Health*. 3rd ed. Burlington, MA: Jones & Bartlett Learning; 2013.

5. Evans AS. Causation and disease: the Henle-Koch postulates revisited. *Yale J Biol Med*. 1976;49(2):175–195.

6. Bradford-Hill A. The environment and disease: association or causation? *Proc R Soc Med*. 1965;58(5):295–300.

7. Oleckno WA. *Essential Epidemiology: Principles and Applications*. 1st ed. Long Grove, IL: Waveland Press; 2002.

8. Centers for Disease Control and Prevention. Vital signs: colorectal cancer screening test use—United States, 2012. *MMWR*. 2013;62(44):881–888.

9. US Department of Health and Human Services. Social determinants of health. Available at: https://www.healthypeople.gov/2020/topics-objectives/topic/social-determinants-of-health. Accessed March 21, 2018.

10. Centers for Disease Control and Prevention. Social determinants of health: know what affects health. Available at: https://www.cdc.gov/socialdeterminants. Accessed May 1, 2017.

11. Rodríguez-Saldaña J. Challenges and opportunities in border health. *Prev Chronic Dis*. 2005;2(1):1–4.

12. Sullivan LM. *Essentials of Biostatistics in Public Health*. 2nd ed. Sudbury, MA: Jones & Bartlett Learning; 2012.

13. Missouri State University. Errors in hypothesis testing. Available at: http://psychstat3. missouristate.edu/Documents/IntroBook3/sbk20.htm. Accessed April 20, 2018.

14. Boston University. Correlation and regression with R. Available at: http://sphweb.bumc. bu.edu/otlt/MPH-Modules/BS/R/R5_Correlation-Regression/NeckCircumference.png. Accessed April 26, 2018.

15. Loi S, Haibe-Kains B, Desmedt C, et al. Predicting prognosis using molecular profiling in estrogen receptor-positive breast cancer treated with tamoxifen. *BMC Genomics*. 2008;9:239.

16. Dembe AE, Partridge JS, Geist LC. Statistical software applications used in health services research: analysis of published studies in the US. *BMC Health Serv Res*. 2011;11(1):252.

2

Communication

Claudia Parvanta, PhD, Alicia Best, PhD, and Vijay Prajapati, BDS, CPH

INTRODUCTION

In public health, communication brings people, messages, and media together in the context of performing prevention, providing health care, and handling emergencies. The Society for Health Communication succinctly describes "health communication" as "[t]he science and art of using communication to advance the health and well-being of people and populations."[1] As the realm of communication can encompass all of our senses, many different types of technologies, and everyday speech, it is even more diffuse than what this definition implies.

The National Communication Association defines communication as, "how people use messages to generate meanings within and across various contexts."[2] Messages, in themselves, represent encoded pieces of information, such as thoughts that are put into words, gestures, glances, and symbols. These messages are shared through a **medium**, such as sound, print, and visual images and are disseminated through a **channel**, such as speaking, radio, magazines, and social media. These components work together so that others perceive what the original sender intended as the meaning. The idea of a source transmitting messages through a channel to a receiver, in anticipation of a response, is a greatly simplified version of the "transactional model of communication."[3] Part of the problem with communication of any kind is that it so rarely works the way we intend. This can be attributable to **noise**, which is anything that interferes with the message being transmitted or received, and then there is the problem with "de-coding" or interpreting the message.

This science of health communication is concerned with improving transmission and interpretation of meaning from one party to another. The tasks in health communication are built upon an evidence base derived from this scientific discipline. We will cover the following health communication tasks in this chapter:

❑ Task 1: Ensure health literacy concepts are applied in communication efforts.
❑ Task 2: Identify communication gaps.
❑ Task 3: Propose recommendations for improving communication processes.
❑ Task 4: Exercise a variety of communication strategies and methods targeting specific populations and venues to promote policies and programs.
❑ Task 5: Communicate effectively and convey information in a manner that is easily understood by diverse audiences (e.g., including persons of limited English proficiency,

those who have low literacy skills or are not literate, individuals with disabilities, and those who are deaf or hard of hearing).

❑ Task 6: Choose communication tools and techniques to facilitate discussions and interactions.

❑ Task 7: Assess the health literacy of populations served.

❑ Task 8: Use risk communication approaches to address public health issues and problems.

❑ Task 9: Set communication goals, objectives, and priorities for a project.

❑ Task 10: Inform the public about health policies, programs, and resources.

❑ Task 11: Apply ethical considerations in developing communication plans and promotional initiatives.

❑ Task 12: Create and disseminate educational information relating to specific emerging health issues and priorities to promote policy development.

❑ Task 13: Communicate the role of public health within the overall health system (e.g., national, state, county, local government) and its impact on the individual.

❑ Task 14: Communicate with colleagues, patients, families, or communities about health disparities and health care disparities.

❑ Task 15: Communicate lessons learned to community partners or global constituencies.

❑ Task 16: Apply facilitation skills in interactions with individuals and groups.

❑ Task 17: Communicate results of population health needs and asset assessments.

❑ Task 18: Communicate with other health professionals in a responsive and responsible manner that supports a team approach to maintaining health of individuals and populations.

❑ Task 19: Provide a rationale for program proposals and evaluations to lay, professional, and policy audiences.

❑ Task 20: Communicate results of evaluation efforts.

Because of the large number of tasks under this domain, we have "chunked" them into 6 clusters. Chunking information is a way to improve the readability of a document. These clusters were developed by the authors and are meant to enhance your comprehension of the material only.

MAJOR CONTENT

Cluster 1: Making Health Communication More Effective

This section describes effective communication strategies, tools, techniques, and media, covering tasks 2, 3, 4, 6, 9, 16, 19, and 20. This systematic application of health communication science to practice was captured first in the National Cancer Institute's (NCI) "Pink Book,"[4] and later in the various versions of the Centers for Disease Control and Prevention's (CDC's) health communication planning tool, *CDCynergy*.[4,5] CDC and NCI were early adopters of a **social marketing** approach, which focuses on the needs and

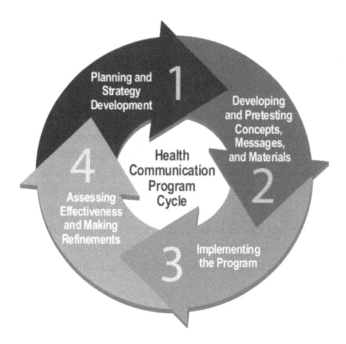

Source: Reprinted from National Cancer Institute.[4]

Figure 2-1. National Cancer Institute's Health Communication Wheel

wants of the intended recipient of the communication.[4,5] Most strategic health communication is based in social marketing's application of commercial marketing and advertising principles to socially beneficial causes.[4,5] We will discuss more about social marketing later in the chapter, but it should not be confused with the practice of using **social media** to sell products. In the same manner that electron microscopes revolutionized biology, we are still learning how to optimize social media platforms for public health communication.[6,7]

The Big Picture

Health communication planning begins in earnest once epidemiologic findings show that a health problem exists and that something can be done to lower exposure or risk. This can be any of a variety of factors, including a change in an environmental condition, a policy, a behavior, or even an attitude that can lead to improvements in health. Health communication can be used to directly instigate or support these changes.

Nearly every health communication treatise references the NCI's health communication process wheel, shown in Figure 2-1[4,8]:

- **Phase 1** generally includes analysis of the problem, the ecological setting, the target population(s), the core intervention strategy, and the partnership mix. Formative research is done at this stage, depending on how much is already known about the problem, the solutions, and the intended recipients of the communication.

- **Phase 2** focuses on developing and producing specific concepts, messages, materials, and media to achieve program objectives. **Pretesting** of procedures and materials with intended users occurs in this phase. With social media platforms, this is no longer a "once-and-done" activity but tends to reiterate throughout the course of a program.

- **Phase 3** requires a tactical plan defining what will be done, when, where, how, and with what money for each piece of the program. Having partners engaged and ready to do their share is essential before the outset of this phase. Once launched, smart programs monitor key performance indicators to make sure the program is on track.

- **Phase 4** leads to assessing the outcomes and impact of the program. This is when results will be published as well as shared through various settings with stakeholders, the public, the media, and so on. As suggested by the wheel shape, the process repeats and what is learned is applied to the next cycle of programming.

The Details

Phase 1 and Phase 2

To move from phase 1 to phase 2 in the planning wheel, health communicators need to be able to answer questions regarding the following topic areas[4,5]:

1. **Audience and objective**: Who are you trying to reach, and what do you want them to do? This is defining the communication gap, presuming the people who need to do something are not aware or motivated to do it.

   In preventive health communication, we define audiences as primary, secondary, and tertiary depending on how close they are to the ones whom you hope will act on the information. The **primary audience** is the individuals you hope will act. A group that potentially has direct and immediate influence over the primary audience is considered a **secondary audience**. Depending upon the primary audience and topic, you might seek out secondary audience figures, such as religious leaders or rock stars. You hope they take up the issue and promote it. A group with indirect influence on the primary audience is called a **tertiary audience**.[9]

2. **The evidence base**: *The Guide to Community Preventive Services* found strong evidence for health communication campaigns that use multiple channels. The guide recommends that one channel must be mass media combined with the distribution of free or reduced-price health-related products.[8] As with all recommendations in *The Community Guide*, a lack of evidence does not mean that an approach does not work—only that there are insufficient publications demonstrating a clear effect. Health communication has also changed somewhat since *The Community Guide* chapter was written in 2009. For example, the *Annual Review of Public Health* published

a "Systematic Review of Reviews" about mobile text messaging for health in 2015.[10] The CDC publishes a selection of studies on a monthly basis that identifies current research as well as points to journals in which such results are published.[11] One should use standard program-planning guidelines to match up the evidence-based approach with one's issue and audience.

3. **Core communication strategy** for each audience: Do you plan to engage a group to create a level of trust and familiarity (e.g., "Hey, we're here, and we want to chat with you.")? Would you like to provide information, but leave their options open, or do you want to try to persuade them to a particular viewpoint or action? The choice of engaging, informing, or persuading determines a great deal of what comes next.

   a. **Engagement** strategies require timely give and take from all parties. Although they may involve in-person clubs and gatherings, they are increasingly moving online through social media. The main goal of engagement is to set up a feeling of mutual understanding. In public health, engagement is a first step toward information or persuasion, unless we truly are providing a forum for others to share their own views, such as on Facebook pages for persons who share a health condition. A question to ask is whether you have the human resources to implement this approach.[5]

   b. **Educational strategies**, or the provision of information, can include framing. **Framing** means presenting information to resonate best with the intended audience. It is important to follow the guidelines used for health literacy and cultural competency (see Chapter 10, "Health Equity and Social Justice") to make information more accessible and meaningful for the intended users.[5]

   c. **Persuasion**: Most public health communication falls into this category, as we really want people to adopt healthy behaviors. We learned a long time ago that just providing information is not enough for 95% of us.[5]

   d. When persuasion is not strong enough, we have **policies**, also known as laws and regulations. These may offer incentives, (e.g., rebates for recycling), or penalties (e.g., fines for noncompliance with car safety seat laws, taxes on tobacco products).[5]

Which Core Communication Strategy Works Best?

Rothschild developed a behavior management approach that compares education, marketing, and policy approaches.[12] While some public health practitioners default to policy (and others to education), there are strengths and weaknesses for each of these approaches.

Educational approaches work best when the recipient of the information has expressed an interest in, or commitment to, the desired behavior. In behavioral economics terms, the costs of doing the recommended behavior appear low and the benefits appear high. For example, most parents are convinced that putting their baby to sleep on its back is safer with little more than information. People who have already been diagnosed with an illness are more likely to follow doctor's instructions than those who are told they can prevent an illness. The **Elaboration Likelihood Model**[13] and the **Health Belief Model** offer explanations of why people are more likely to respond well to information when they feel they are more susceptible or already have an illness condition.[14]

Regulatory or policy approaches are necessary when the perceived costs of adopting a behavior are high, and the benefits appear low. For example, many motorcycle riders prefer the freedom of not wearing a helmet—state helmet laws are necessary to prevent more head injuries and deaths. Many parents might forgo child safety seats because of the costs, inconvenience, and mistaken belief they can hold their child safely in their arms. Again, laws are necessary to protect innocent lives. The way to get new policies created is through grass roots efforts and other communication strategies that build up a demand among policymakers to address their constituents' needs.

For everything in between (i.e., where the cost and benefit can be negotiated), there is social marketing. **Social marketing** uses the term **product** to refer to a tangible good, such as soap, a condom, or a vegetable. It also uses the term *product* to refer to services (e.g., Special Supplemental Nutrition Program for Women, Infants, and Children; Supplemental Nutrition Assistance Program), or behavioral suggestions (e.g., washing your hands before meals, using a condom, eating more vegetables). The social marketer researches what the intended user would value in the new product compared with what products they are presently using or what behaviors they are presently performing. The goal of social marketing is to raise the value of the new product relative to the old, and this can be done by adjusting the so-called **four Ps of marketing**: the product's **price**, in terms of time, money, and other consumer values; **place,** or physical location; its positioning or how the consumer sees the **product** serving his or her needs; and the **promotional strategy**. As an example, Andreasen's benchmark criteria for social marketing have been embraced by most practitioners and form the basis for curricular competencies in social marketing.[15]

Phase 3: Rounding out the Communication Plan

Is communication the primary intervention or is it supporting other strategies? In other words, are you offering services or products and using communication to promote their uptake, or are you trying to change behavior through communication alone?[5] Other questions you might need to answer are as follows:

- What settings and modalities are at your disposal? Are you working one-on-one, with a group, or with mass media? What communication vehicles do you plan to use?
- Is the exchange taking place in person, in real time (possibly through digital channels), or through some recorded, symbolic interaction (print, video, or other form of non–real-time transmission)?
- How much time do you have?

- How much money do you have?
- How many people do you have to do the work?

Answering these questions generates a macro plan that guides the rest of a strategic communication intervention.

Phase 4: Evaluation

As mentioned previously, formative and process evaluation takes place during phases 1 through 3. By this stage, you would have created and pretested your messages and materials (formative stage) and determined that they were being disseminated as planned (process stage). In outcome evaluation, one is generally testing whether exposure to the communication campaign results in the desired behavior change or results in the desired precursor to behavior change, such as knowledge acquisition or attitude change.

Evaluation in health communication is similar to other forms of program evaluation (see Chapter 7, "Program Planning and Evaluation") in that it begins with engaging stakeholders and determining what metrics will count. During the evaluation, you are answering three questions: Are you doing the right things? Are you doing the right things right? And are you doing enough of the right things to make a difference?[16] Finally, you need to be able to measure the change, creating a fourth question. Communication interventions have some unique characteristics that line up with the four questions:

1. **Doing the right things?** The evidence base for health communication interventions is growing. In addition to the previously mentioned *The Community Guide*, researchers have used program-tested specific archives such as NCI's Research-Tested Intervention Programs[17] or CDC's best practices for HIV prevention[18] and so on. Health communication programs that adhere to a behavior change theory and design interventions that operationalize its constructs (e.g., an intervention using social cognitive theory might strive to build self-efficacy, provide vicarious learning, or demonstrate rewards) are stronger because they are built on logic models of how and why change is predicted. This logic model is the framework for program evaluation.

   "Doing the right things" also means being mindful of local community standards. We know that tailoring messages to specific audiences is more effective than "one size fits all." For example, language and imagery that work well for adolescents or individuals who define themselves as LGBTQ might be offensive to others in the community. It is important to offer community leaders the opportunity to review and comment on materials and try to engage them in understanding the necessity of tailoring or targeting communications. There have been excellent examples of framing to position messages to be effective and acceptable to the community at large.[1,19]

2. **Doing the right things right?** Maintaining the quality of a communication program involves careful coordination and monitoring of content dissemination across all chan-

nels. These days, Web site analytics reports or media tracking services can provide accurate counts of **impressions**, the term for exposure of content on a channel, such as print ads or TV spots.[20] With interpersonal communications, training and fidelity monitoring is more of a challenge as it depends on individual personalities and other human factors. Many public health communication campaigns include a call to action to go to a hotline or, increasingly, a social media site. These need to be staffed and the content constantly updated to maintain audience involvement.

3. **Doing enough to make a difference?** The third question regards whether enough of the target audience heard or saw the message to be able to detect the prespecified difference. Robert Hornik, a frequently cited health communication evaluation expert, found that the largest error in health communication campaigns is inadequate **reach**, with often less than 50% of the intended audience receiving the message.[21] The next question is related to **dose** and, frankly, there is no known threshold for this. For some people, hearing a message once will change their mind forever about an issue. Others need to go through all the stages of change (i.e., precontemplation, contemplation, trial, repetition, maintenance) and receive different forms of communication to move from one stage to the next.

4. **Can you tell?** Finally, as is true for all evaluations, a large enough sample is necessary to detect the difference. Health communication interventions do well when they see a 15-percentage-point change generally measured within a year of program onset.[22,23]

Interpersonal Communication

Tasks 6 and 16 deal with ways to improve one-on-one or group communication. Task 6 focuses on making you a better listener and partner in an exchange, while task 16 emphasizes your group facilitation skills. Nearly every college or university requires students to take a Communication 101 course that lays out the principles of effective listening, thinking, and speaking. **Patient-centeredness** is a defining principle that places the patient's needs and abilities at the heart of any communication encounter, whether in clinical or public health. The NCI illustrates the six core functions of patient–clinician communication that affect health outcomes, as shown in Figure 2-2.

There are tools to improve communication that support each of these nodes. You are encouraged to explore the Academy of Communication in Healthcare for training and resources pertaining to patient–provider communication.[25]

In terms of assessing skills, the Roter Interaction Analysis System (or RIAS) allows a trained observer to code interactions of health care providers and patients.[26] This gold standard has been used in hundreds of published studies worldwide.

Group facilitation is a special talent that needs to be taken seriously. In principle, it requires applying the respect and active listening skills you would use in a conversation with your best friend to a group. The Community Tool Box has a useful set of tips for how to keep a group on task, on agenda, and in harmony.[27]

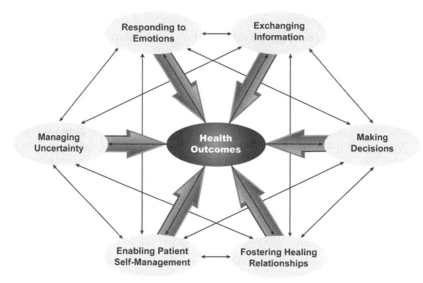

Source: Reprinted from National Institutes of Health.[24]
Figure 2-2. Six Core Functions of Patient–Clinician Communication

Cluster 2: Health Literacy and Cultural Tasks in Health Communication

Consistent with the focus of *Healthy People 2020*, three tasks deal with **health literacy** (tasks 1, 5, and 7).[28] In addition, it makes sense to also include "culturally competent health communication" in this skill set. There are numerous resources to support these activities, including the National Standards for Culturally and Linguistically Appropriate Services in Health and Health Care (CLAS Standards),[29] the CDC's Clear Communication Index,[30] and Boston University's Health Literacy Tool Shed.[31]

The US government defines health literacy as "the degree to which individuals can obtain, process, understand, and communicate about health-related information needed to make informed health decisions."[32] There are several frameworks that lay out the determinants, applications, and outcomes for health literacy. Sørensen et al. and Squiers et al. provide clear examples of such frameworks.[33,34] Poor health literacy is both a cause and a consequence of other health disparities, resulting in needless suffering and billions of dollars of wasted resources. For this reason, the Affordable Care Act (ACA) has several health literacy measures and mandates.[35] The Plain Writing Act of 2010[36] requires federal agencies to use clear language so that citizens may "[f]ind what they need, understand what they find; and use what they find to meet their needs."[37]

The National Action Plan to Improve Health Literacy provides goals and strategies to simplify and decode all health information for nearly everyone. Health literacy is also context-specific or, in other words, people process information differently depending upon where they are receiving it. Those visiting a doctor are likely to be sick and/or stressed. The noise and distractions in most markets or drugstores add to the burden of a reader. Keeping these factors in mind, it is important to recognize that at some time or another, all of us will need clear health information. CDC's Clear Communication Index (CCI) is an assessment tool that can be applied to any print material to determine not only its readability level but also to what extent it conveys information that is compelling and actionable.[30] Readability of documents, which is essentially measuring word length, can be assessed by using the Flesch-Kincaid Grade Level Readability Test or SMOG (Simple Measure of Gobbledygook), which are included in Microsoft Word. The CCI, however, offers more sophisticated approaches to readability.

As defined previously, health literacy involves comprehension of English, as a first or second language; the ability to read tables, charts, or other graphical displays; and a general understanding of health concepts. Because of the sensitivities that most people feel about demonstrating their abilities to read or not, assessing an individual's literacy level is not something that should be done routinely. But, there are times when such assessment is necessary. For example, in a medical setting, if certain patients are comfortable with the Internet, they can be directed to online resources. Alternatively, they might better understand simple print materials or need everything in an audiovisual form. Any of these media might need to be produced in a different language for users.

Assessments used in research include the Rapid Estimate of Adult Literacy in Medicine (REALM)[38] and the Test of Functional Health Literacy in Adults (TOFHLA).[39] The Newest Vital Sign,[40] the Numeracy Understanding in Medicine Instrument (NUmi),[41] and the eHealth Literacy Scale (eHEALS)[42] were designed more for clinical practice. The approach that practitioners are urged to take is one of **universal precautions**, in that understanding should be confirmed with everyone, and no one should be placed in a situation in which they feel uncomfortable or judged. The Agency for Healthcare Research and Quality has created a Universal Precautions Toolkit. A primary communication tool for confirming understanding is called "teach back."[43,44]

Cluster 3: Risk Communication

There is only one task in this group, but it is a big one. Risk communication (task 8) can occur in many different environments. It can occur in the calm, quiet space of a doctor's office while he or she is comparing the probabilities of success of two procedures. An environmental health agent may need to present the potential **hazards** of living near a nuclear power plant and what citizens can do as preventive measures. The most challenging aspect of risk communication, however, takes place during a disaster of natural or human creation. As a public health official, you can prepare yourself and your team to communicate effectively during a crisis. The CDC has a training program and free resource to guide you in this area,[45] much of it based on the work of Covello[46] and Sandman.[47]

Hazard, risk, exposure, and causality are all seemingly straightforward terms. The US Environmental Protection Agency (EPA) has some excellent tools to explain these concepts[48] but, in brief, a **hazard** is a source of potential damage or harm, **exposure** is contact with the hazard, and **risk** is the probability that a person will be harmed by this exposure. Hill's criteria are commonly used to assess the strength of an argument for **causality**.[49] Much of what we learned about communicating about risk to populations has been derived from the experience of the EPA and the Agency for Toxic Substance and Disease Registry (ATSDR),[50] as well as its sister agency, CDC. Before September 11, 2001, and the anthrax attacks, there had not been extensive communication about exposure and risk outside of natural disasters and environmental contamination. However, after the events of 9/11, we had to become conversant in emergency risk communication (see Chapter 5, "Public Health Biology and Human Disease Risk").

Disaster Management

The new millennium brought an exponential focus on communication in emergencies and, in particular, providing information to the exposed, first responders, and concentric circles of audiences. Also reached were individuals considered not to be at risk, but who worried about those who were. This configuration of audiences is one primary distinction between

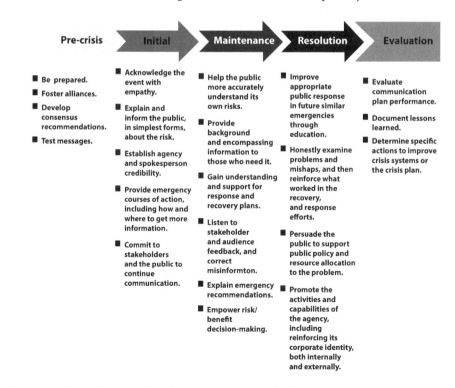

Source: Adapted from Centers for Disease Control and Prevention (CDC).[45]

Figure 2-3. CDC's Crisis and Emergency Communication Planning Cycle

Table 2-1. Sample Message Map for Avian Flu

What Is Avian Flu?		
Key Message 1	**Key Message 2**	**Key Message 3**
Avian flu is normally found in birds.	It's possible for avian flu to spread to humans.	An outbreak is possible.
Supporting Fact 1-1	**Supporting Fact 2-1**	**Supporting Fact 3-1**
A form of avian flu is widespread in Asia.	Avian flu rarely affects humans.	Disease can be spread from country to country.
Supporting Fact 1-2	**Supporting Fact 2-2**	**Supporting Fact 3-2**
Avian flu outbreaks in the United States have been successfully contained.	The bird virus could combine with human virus to spread more easily.	Plans are being developed to produce vaccine quickly.
Supporting Fact 1-3	**Supporting Fact 2-3**	**Supporting Fact 3-3**
The United States is strengthening surveillance to identify disease.	Avian flu can cause serious disease and death.	Antiviral drugs will be stockpiled.

emergency communication and other forms of health communication. The main message for emergency communication is to plan for its inevitable occurrence. Figure 2-3 shows a cycle recommended by the CDC in its Crisis and Emergency Communication training manual.

A key tool used to plan for emergencies is Covello's "Message Maps." These Message Maps allow everyone charged with sharing information to work in sync. Messages are presented in three short messages in fewer than 27 words each. This is approximately equal to one "sound bite" in typical broadcast media.[45] Table 2-1 is a sample Message Map showing three main messages and supporting information for Avian influenza.

Moving away from public health emergencies, risk communication is also part of standard health and medical communication, whether one is getting an immunization, receiving a routine procedure such as a mammogram, or considering surgery or alternatives. **Shared decision-making** is the goal of medicine these days. For patients to truly participate in decisions concerning treatment choices, they need to understand the meaning of risks and probabilities—an area that is difficult for many patients regardless of educational level. **Decision aids** are used to contextualize and explain these abstract concepts.[51] The International Patient Decision Aids Standards Collaboration publishes and reviews criteria for effective aids.[52,53] In addition, the best health care providers use touch, eye contact, and, above all, listening carefully, to enhance interpersonal communication.

Cluster 4: Nonemergency Communication

Tasks here deal with **nonemergency communication** of specific kinds of information to the public, including health policies, programs, resources, emerging health issues, the role of public health, and the results of evaluations (tasks 10, 12, 13, and 20). Skills in this area include communicating with the media as well as preparation of information directly for the public. The National Public Health Information Coalition provides many useful resources to this end.[54]

This cluster represents the everyday function of most public information officers, in any public health–related setting. According to Nelson, "it is important to consider what audiences want from experts in public health and other areas. From a communication perspective, most people want to know answers to the following questions."[55] Nelson proceeds to list the questions necessary for nonemergency communication[55]:

- What did you find? (Description)
- Why did it happen? (Explanation)
- What does it mean? (Interpretation)
- What needs to be done about it? (Action)[55]

These four key questions are useful when one is constructing information about the results of a study or evaluation, an emerging public health issue (e.g., the opioid epidemic), a policy or program, or the role of public health in general.

The CDC's media relations office developed a tool for scientists to use when publishing studies that were going to be released to the public, the "Single Overriding Communication Objective" or SOCO form.[56,57] This forces authors to present their information in one paragraph, to list three key facts that they want the audience to remember, and to provide a main message. Although a Message Map is used primarily when one is addressing a live audience, the SOCO helps anyone sharing information with any media channel (e.g., press reporters, radio, TV) be accurate and consistent with their message.

Most of the time in public health we feel we need to share numbers with the public. This can be challenging because of the relative lack of **"health numeracy"** of the average individual. The most recent major survey of the US public from the Program for the International Assessment of Adult Competencies found that 64% of individuals between the ages of 16 and 65 years who participated in the survey were in the lower three levels of the five-level numeracy scale. They iterated that "6 out of 10 adults in the United States are unlikely to be able to add up a total amount payable for shoes on sale for 'buy one pair, get a second pair of equal or lesser value for half price,' given the price for each pair."[58]

It is clear that even the most educated people can get bogged down in information overload, particularly when it comes to many numbers. The best advice is to use data sparingly, use whole numbers, explain unfamiliar terms, and choose visualization tools carefully. Numbers rarely speak for themselves, and when they do, most people will get them wrong. Figure 2-4 shows a sample numerical infographic.

Cluster 5: Professional Communication

This cluster features largely **professional communication**, such as when sharing information with state and local colleagues, health care professionals, community-based organizations, and others whom we see as partners, about health disparities, programmatic

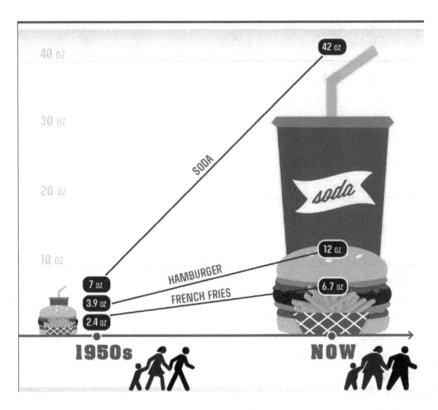

Source: Reprinted from Centers for Disease Control and Prevention.[59]

Figure 2-4. Sample Numerical Infographic

lessons learned, population needs assessments, health care, and seeking new resources through proposals (tasks 14, 15, 17, 18, and 19). Organizations such as the Association of State and Territorial Health Officials (ASTHO),[60] the National Association of City and County Health Officials (NACCHO),[61] the American Public Health Association (APHA),[62] and the Association of Schools and Programs of Public Health (ASPPH)[63] provide models for how this is done. In addition, many government agencies serve as conduits of information to specific health care partners, such as the Health Resources and Services Administration (HRSA),[64] which works with federally qualified health centers across the country. The Surgeon General's reports[65] and *Morbidity and Mortality Weekly Report* (*MMWR*)[66] set standards in this area.

This area comprises many specific forms of communication but, in this case, you are communicating with other professionals, generally in a nonemergency context. We emphasized the need to minimize data and make things as clear and simple as possible when communicating with the public (cluster 4). The need for clarity and simplicity applies to communicating with professional colleagues, except this cluster emphasizes sharing data in many forms, explaining the results of studies and assessments, disseminating clinical or policy guidelines, or collaborating on proposals for programmatic funding. An excellent reference for this task is Nelson et al., *Making Data Talk*.[67] See the following related information about communication resources.

Health Disparities

The US government has gradually moved from a focus on reducing health disparities to achieving health equity and the elimination of disparities in our 10-year goals, defined in *Healthy People*. An obvious place where communication competency in this area is required is in the preparation of the Office of Minority Health's Annual Health Disparities and Inequalities Report.[68]

Programmatic Lessons Learned

The *Guide to Community Preventive Services*, NCI's Cancer PLANET, HIV-AIDS Programs that Work, and the Patient Centered Outcomes Research Institute (PCORI) are all examples of ways to communicate about programmatic lessons learned. These all include versions for professional and lay readers alike. The bar for evidence-based interventions is quite high these days. The primary route to becoming part of the evidence base is to publish clinical trials and other intervention studies in peer-reviewed journals.

Population Needs Assessments

Population needs assessments are done through surveys of local to national populations. Examples of such surveys include the Behavior Risk Factor Surveillance System (BRFSS), the National Health and Nutrition Examination Survey (NHANES), or the Health Information National Trends Survey (HINTS). Also, data can be obtained from surveillance systems of other reported events, such as births, deaths, pregnancy, and notifiable diseases, which are often combined with questionnaires (e.g., Pregnancy Risk Assessment Monitoring System [PRAMS]).

There are multiple accepted ways to share the results. The BRFSS presents a range of documents that break out findings by population or topic. You can see that some of these are meant for policy or public readers, whereas others anticipate a public health or medically trained reader (e.g., *MMWR* reports of findings). The CDC's National Center for Health Statistics publishes an annual report entitled, "Health, United States," which compiles data from across federal agencies. In addition, it focuses on specific topics each year (such as health disparities) and shows data trends for major indicators. Finally, many states and even counties have chosen to work with *The Guide to Community Preventive Services* (https://www.thecommunityguide.org) to select interventions with good evidence of effectiveness.

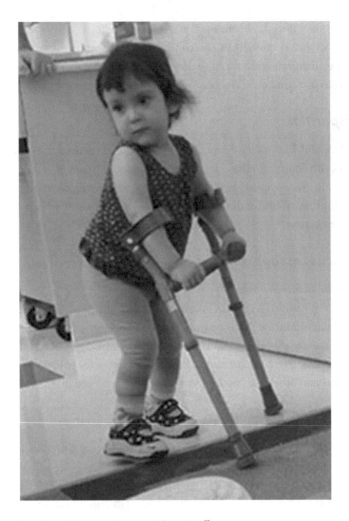

Source: Reprinted from Centers for Disease Control and Prevention.[69]

Figure 2-5. Child With Spina Bifida

Cluster 6: Ethics in Health Communication

In this cluster there is only a single task (task 11), which charges us to do everything mentioned previously in an ethical manner. Using health communication in an ethical manner adheres closely to the guidelines set forth in Chapter 4, "Law and Ethics."

As intermediaries between public health authorities and audiences, including health care practitioners, the media, and the public, our primary responsibility is to ensure accuracy of information and to attempt to provide information that all of the audience can understand. This can be considered part of our professional ethical code. Health communicators face ethical dilemmas when what might be the best way to present information to one audience segment, such as using words or graphics that appeal to that audience, might be harmful to another. For example, CDC and the March of Dimes did extensive testing of materials to explain the connection between neural tube defects, including spina bifida, and inadequate intake of folic acid before conception. In focus group after focus group, women asked that pictures of children born with highly disfiguring conditions (such as those born without closure of the skull and the brain bulging through) be shown so that "women would understand the seriousness" of the condition. Even though women thought these somewhat shocking materials would make the point effectively, the health communication team chose to use pictures portraying children who were alive and otherwise healthy in their print materials (see Figure 2-5). How would you interpret this decision through an ethical lens?

PRACTICE QUESTIONS

Vignette 1: *In planning a smoking prevention program for youth, the health communicator at the YMCA asked to speak to the Parents and Teachers Association of the nearby school, restaurant owners, and sports coaches. She hoped that they would support a local ban on smoking near or around any outdoor space where children played or ate.*

1. Which audience group was she focusing on to launch her program?
    a. Primary audience—the teens and children themselves
    b. Secondary audience—the parents and teachers of the kids
    c. Tertiary audience—creating a community norm and policy endorsement
    d. A combination of a and b
    e. A combination of b and c

Answer: e. Both the secondary and tertiary audience. Think about why it makes sense to start with these groups rather than the teenagers directly.

Vignette 2: *A state health department has detected a disparity in infant mortality across its multiple counties. The eight counties with the highest infant mortality rates are diverse regarding socioeconomic status, race/ethnicity, and geography. Five of the target counties are in rural parts of the state, while the other three counties are located in more urban areas. You are a member of this interdisciplinary team tasked with developing a health communication intervention to address this problem.*

2. One behavior identified by the team developing the intervention is the primary risk factor for infant death, co-sleeping (i.e., parents sharing the same bed with baby). In a health communication campaign to address co-sleeping, who is considered the primary audience?
    a. Parents of infants
    b. Pregnant women
    c. Pediatricians and obstetricians–gynecologists
    d. Celebrities

Answer: a. A primary audience is the decision-maker, whereas the secondary audience is the one influencing the primary audience. In this case, the target group for the behavior change is the parents of an infant who would eventually avoid the practice of co-sleeping. The secondary audience would be the pediatricians and the obstetricians–gynecologists who would influence or rather educate the parents about the harmful effects of co-sleeping. The celebrities would be the tertiary audience as they can promote safe sleeping habits and indirectly influence the parents.

3. You are tasked with engaging the target population in your team's efforts to address infant mortality in each county. Which of the following best describes an engagement strategy?
    a. Conducting focus groups with women of child-bearing age
    b. Distributing educational material about infant mortality through magazines and flyers at places frequently visited by young women
    c. Hosting a Facebook page for parents to discuss their experiences with breastfeeding
    d. Advocating policy related to access to health care for pregnant women

Answer: c. Engagement refers to creating a level of trust and familiarity toward individuals *before* informing or attempting to persuade. Hence, social media platforms open group discussions and are ideal for creating a familiar medium to share ideas. Conducting focus groups is a targeted approach for research. Educating and policymaking do not fall into the category of engagement either.

4. Which of the following is a common metric used to evaluate health communication?
    a. Number reached
    b. Frequency of exposure
    c. Next day recall of message
    d. All of the above

Answer: d. Each of these options can be used to evaluate a health communication campaign. To adequately evaluate health communication, you should track the extent to which your target audience remembers seeing or hearing your message (recall and reach), as well as how many times they were exposed to it (dose). These metrics can help attribute results to your campaign.

Vignette 3: *The CDC has developed a generic brochure to promote colorectal cancer screening. It features primarily white models. You run it through a Flesch-Kincaid screener and find it reads at a 12th-grade level.*

5. How would you adapt this material to be the most useful in general? What would you do to adapt it for non–English-speaking Hispanic women in your community?

Sample response: Different approaches can be used to assess the best methods for conveying colorectal cancer screening information. Focus groups, individual interviews, and surveys can be used to collect data to assess the health literacy of the populations and assess how they are understanding communication materials. Specifically, you may administer a brief health literacy assessment tool to a representative sample of the target population and then adjust the reading level of your materials to align with the average health literacy level of the sample. In general, materials should be written at a 7th-grade reading level as this reflects the majority of American adults. You may also conduct a series of pretesting focus groups in which you examine how your messages are being perceived and understood by the target population.

Additional information: Examples of health literacy measurement tools include the Short Assessment of Health Literacy–Spanish and English, consist of comparable tests in English and Spanish, and have good reliability and validity in both languages. This tests the individual's comprehension as well as pronunciation (decoding) of health-related terms. Administration of the test takes only 2 to 3 minutes and requires minimal training.

The Rapid Estimate of Adult Literacy in Medicine—Short Form (REALM-SF) is a seven-item word-recognition test to provide clinicians with a valid quick assessment of patient health literacy. The REALM-SF has been validated and field tested in diverse research settings and has excellent agreement with the 66-item REALM instrument in terms of grade-level assignments.

6. What strategy may be used to develop effective communication materials for populations with low health literacy?
   a. Engage members of the target population in the message development process.
   b. Take a "universal precautions" approach to message design.
   c. Use targeted or tailored rather than generic materials.
   d. All of the above

Answer: d. Engaging the population is the first step in developing a level of trust. Similarly, taking a universal precautions approach will avoid any judgments on the part of participants who would tend to be more uncomfortable because of their low health literacy status. Using targeted materials based on literacy level and cultural and other demographic characteristics can help facilitate a more accurate, efficient, and faster process for citizens to "find what they need, understand what they find; and use what they find to meet their needs."[37]

7. What is a key principle to consider when developing and assessing health communication messages?
   a. Reading level
   b. Text density
   c. Use of jargon
   d. All of the above

Answer: d. All of the above factors are key components in deciding the health literacy level of your target population and adjusting your messages accordingly.

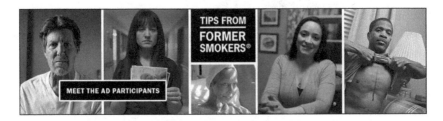

Source: Reprinted from Centers for Disease Control and Prevention.[70]

Figure 2-6. Tips From Former Smokers Campaign

Vignette 4: *The "Tips from Former Smokers Campaign" features living, and now some deceased, individuals sharing their thoughts on how to cope with disabilities and illnesses they attribute to their smoking. The ads are quite graphic and emphasize the suffering of real people who participated in the ads (see Figure 2-6).*

8. How would you interpret the ethics decision that the CDC had to make in order to use this approach?

Sample response: One ethics consideration is related to informed consent. Before moving forward with development and implementation of the campaign, CDC should be sure that participants are fully informed about how their images would be portrayed and how broadly the ads would be shared. Also, CDC should consider participants' family members and to what extent they should be allowed to participate in the decision-making process. In addition, the initial stages of campaign development should include adequate pretesting to avoid potential ethical dilemmas down the road. For example, pretesting is essential to ensure materials do not cause unintended consequences such as embarrassment and mockery to participants and their families.

CONCLUSION

In this chapter, we broadly covered communication tasks, clustering competencies into groups. Communication is central to public health as suggested by its representation as a cross-cutting skill, as well as a special area of study. As said by Rimal and Lapinski, communication is at the heart of who we are as human beings. It is our way of exchanging information and it also signifies our symbolic capability. Also, as researchers and practitioners from diverse disciplines come together and adopt multilevel theoretical approaches, there is a clear role for health communication to be an important driver in providing input and saving lives.[71]

REFERENCES

1. Society for Health Communcation. Redefining health communication. Available at: https://shc.memberclicks.net/our-activities. Accessed March 12, 2018.

2. National Communication Association. What is communication? Available at: https://www. natcom.org/about-nca/what-communication. Accessed March 12, 2018.

3. Barnlund DC. Transactional model of communication. In: Sereno KK, Mortensen CD, eds. *Foundations of Communication Theory*. New York, NY: Harper & Row; 1970:99.

4. National Cancer Institute. Making health communication programs work. US Department of Health and Human Services. 2002. Available at: https://www.cancer.gov/publications/ health-communication/pink-book.pdf. Accessed March 12, 2018.

5. Centers for Disease Control and Prevention. CDCynergy Web: Your guide to effective health communication. Available at: https://www.orau.gov/cdcynergy/web. Accessed March 13, 2018.

6. Parvanta CF, Nelson DE, Harner RN. *Public Health Communication: Critical Tools and Strategies*. 1st ed. Burlington, MA: Jones & Bartlett Learning; 2017.

7. Harrington NG. *Health Communication: Theory, Method and Application*. 1st ed. New York, NY: Routledge; 2014.

8. Elder RW; Community Preventive Services Task Force. Combination of mass media health campaigns and health-related product distribution is recommended to improve healthy behaviors. *Am J Prev Med*. 2014;47(3):372–374.

9. Parvanta CF. A public health communication planning framework. In: Parvanta CF, Nelson DE, Harner RN, eds. *Public Health Commuication: Critical Tools and Strategies*. Burlington, MA: Jones & Bartlett Learning; 2017:47–48.

10. Hall AK, Cole-Lewis H, Bernhardt JM. Mobile text messaging for health: a systematic review of reviews. *Annu Rev Public Health*. 2015;36(1):393–415.

11. Centers for Disease Control and Prevention. Health communication science digest. Available at: www.cdc.gov/healthcommunication/sciencedigest/index.html. Accessed March 19, 2018.

12. Rothschild ML. Carrots, sticks, and promises: a conceptual framework for the management of public health and social issue behaviors. *J Mark*. 1999;63(4):24–37.

13. National Cancer Institute. Theory at a glance: a guide for health promotion practice. National Institutes of Health. 2005. Available at: https://cancercontrol.cancer.gov/brp/ research/theories_project/theory.pdf. Accessed June 13, 2018.

14. Glanz K, Rimer BK, Viswanath K. *Health Behavior: Theory, Research, and Practice*. 5th ed. San Francisco, CA: Jossey-Bass; 2015.

15. Andreasen AR. Marketing social marketing in the social change marketplace. *J Public Policy Mark*. 2002;21(1):3–13.

16. Kennedy MG, DeShazo J. Evaluating a health communication program. In: Parvanta CF, Nelson DE, Harner RN, eds. *Public Health Communication: Critical Tools and Strategies*. 1st ed. Burlington, MA: Jones & Bartlett Learning; 2017:369–390.

17. National Cancer Institute. Research-tested intervention programs (RTIPs). Available at: https://rtips.cancer.gov/rtips/index.do. Accessed March 19, 2018.

18. Centers for Disease Control and Prevention. Compendium of evidence-based interventions and best practices for HIV prevention. Available at: https://www.cdc.gov/hiv/research/interventionresearch/compendium/index.html. Accessed March 19, 2018.

19. Kirby SD, Robinson SJ. Framing messages about sexual health: research for engaging all stakeholders. In: Parvanta CF, Nelson DE, Harner RN, eds. *Public Health Commuication: Critical Tools and Strategies.* 1st ed. Burlington, MA: Jones & Bartlett Learning; 2017:251–264.

20. Centers for Disease Control and Prevention. CDC social media tools, guidelines & best practices. Available at: https://www.cdc.gov/SocialMedia/Tools/guidelines/index.html. Accessed March 19, 2018.

21. Hornik RC. *Public Health Communication: Evidence for Behavior Change.* Mahwah, NJ: Lawrence Erlbaum Associates; 2002.

22. Snyder LB, Hamilton MA, Mitchell EW, Kiwanuka-Tondo J, Fleming-Milici F, Proctor D. A meta-analysis of the effect of mediated health communication campaigns on behavior change in the United States. *J Health Commun.* 2004;9(S1):71–96.

23. Noar SM, Pierce LB, Black HG. Can computer-mediated interventions change theoretical mediators of safer sex? A meta-analysis. *Hum Commun Res.* 2010;36(3):261–297.

24. Epstein RM, Street RL Jr. *Patient-Centered Communication in Cancer Care: Promoting Healing and Reducing Suffering.* Bethesda, MD: National Institutes of Health; 2007.

25. Academy of Communication in Healthcare. Better communication. Better relationships. Better care. Available at: https://www.achonline.org. Accessed March 19, 2018.

26. Roter D, Larson S. The Roter Interaction Analysis System (RIAS): utility and flexibility for analysis of medical interactions. *Patient Educ Couns.* 2002;46(4):243–251.

27. Center for Community Health and Development at the University of Kansas. Section 2. Developing facilitation skills. Available at: http://ctb.ku.edu/en/table-of-contents/leadership/group-facilitation/facilitation-skills/main. Accessed March 19, 2018.

28. Office of Disease Prevention and Health Promotion. Health communication and health information technology. Available at: https://www.healthypeople.gov/2020/topics-objectives/topic/health-communication-and-health-information-technology. Accessed March 19, 2018.

29. US Department of Health and Human Services Office of Minority Health. The national CLAS standards. Available at: https://minorityhealth.hhs.gov/omh/browse.aspx?lvl=2&lvlid=53. Accessed March 20, 2018.

30. Centers for Disease Control and Prevention. Clear communication index user guide. Available at: https://www.cdc.gov/ccindex/tool. Accessed March 20, 2018.

31. Boston University. Health literacy tool shed. Available at: https://healthliteracy.bu.edu. Accessed March 20, 2018.

32. Berkman ND, Davis TC, McCormack L. Health literacy: what is it? *J Health Commun.* 2010;15(suppl 2):9–19.

33. Sørensen K, Van den Broucke S, Fullam J, et al. Health literacy and public health: a systematic review and integration of definitions and models. *BMC Public Health.* 2012;12(1):80.

34. Squiers L, Peinado S, Berkman N, Boudewyns V, McCormack L. The health literacy skills framework. *J Health Commun.* 2012;17(suppl 3):30–54.

35. Somers SA, Mahadevan R. Health literacy implications of the Affordable Care Act. Center for Health Care Strategies. 2010. Available at: https://www.chcs.org/media/Health_Literacy_ Implications_of_the_Affordable_Care_Act.pdf. Accessed June 13, 2018.

36. Plain Writing Act of 2010, 5 USC § 301 note (2010).

37. US Department of Health and Human Services, US Food and Drug Administration. Federal plain language guidelines. Available at: https://www.fda.gov/AboutFDA/PlainLanguage/ ucm346268.htm. Accessed March 20, 2018.

38. Davis T, Long S, Jackson R, et al. Rapid estimate of adult literacy in medicine: a shortened screening instrument. *Fam Med.* 1993;25(6):391–395.

39. Parker R, Baker D, Williams M, Nurss J. The test of functional health literacy in adults: a new instrument for measuring patients' literacy skills. *J Gen Intern Med.* 1995;10(10):537–541.

40. Pfizer. The newest vital sign. Available at: https://www.pfizer.com/health/literacy/public- policy-researchers/nvs-toolkit. Accessed March 20, 2018.

41. Schapira MM, Walker CM, Cappaert KJ, et al. The Numeracy Understanding in Medicine Instrument: a measure of health numeracy developed using item response theory. *Med Decis Making.* 2012;32(6):851–865.

42. Norman CD, Skinner HA. eHEALS: The eHealth literacy scale. *J Med Internet Res.* 2006; 8(4):e27.

43. US Department of Health and Human Services, Agency for Healthcare Research and Quality. Health literacy universal precautions toolkit, 2nd edition. Use the teach-back method: tool #5. Available at: https://www.ahrq.gov/professionals/quality-patient-safety/quality-resources/tools/ literacy-toolkit/healthlittoolkit2-tool5.html. Accessed March 20, 2018.

44. Hedden EM. Health literacy and clear health communication. In: Parvanta CF, Nelson DE, Harner RN, eds. *Public Health Commuication: Critical Tools and Strategies.* 1st ed. Burlington, MA: Jones & Bartlett Learning; 2017:1.

45. Centers for Disease Control and Prevention. Emergency preparedness and response. Available at: https://emergency.cdc.gov/cerc/resources. Accessed March 20, 2018.

46. Covello VT. Best practices in public health risk and crisis communication. *J Health Commun.* 2003;8(suppl 1):5–8.

47. Sandman PM. The Peter M. Sandman risk communication website. Available at: http://www. psandman.com. Accessed March 20, 2018.

48. US Environmental Protection Agency. Risk assessment guidance for superfund (RAGS): Part A. Available at: https://www.epa.gov/risk/risk-assessment-guidance-superfund-rags-part. Accessed March 20, 2018.

49. Bradford-Hill A. The environment and disease: association or causation? *Proc R Soc Med.* 1965;58(5):295–300.

50. Agency for Toxic Substances and Disease Registry. Available at: https://www.atsdr.cdc.gov. Accessed March 20, 2018.

51. Elwyn G, O'Connor A, Stacey D, Volk R, Edwards A, Coulter A. Developing a quality criteria framework for patient decision aids: online international delphi consensus process. *BMJ.* 2006;333(7565):417–419.

52. Drug and Therapeutics Bulletin. An introduction to patient decision aids. *BMJ.* 2013; 346(f4147):1–4.

53. International Patient Decision Aid Standards (IPDAS) Collaboration. Available at: http:// ipdas.ohri.ca. Accessed May 3, 2018.

54. National Public Health Information Coalition. Available at: https://www.nphic.org. Accessed March 20, 2018.

55. Nelson DE. Public health communication. In: Parvanta CF, Nelson DE, Harner RN, eds. *Public Health Communication: Critical Tools and Strategies.* Burlington, MA: Jones & Bartlett Learning; 2017:104.

56. Centers for Disease Control and Prevention. Sample single overriding communications objective (SOCO). Available at: https://www.cdc.gov/tb/publications/guidestoolkits/forge/docs/13_samplesingleoverridingcommunicationsobjective_soco_worksheet.doc. Accessed May 3, 2018.

57. Howard RJ. Getting it right in prime time: tools and strategies for media interaction. *Emerg Infect Dis.* 2000;6(4):426–427.

58. Program for the International Assessment of Adult Competencies. PIAAC: What the data say about the skills of US adults. Available at: https://static1.squarespace.com/static/51bb74b8 e4b0139570ddf020/t/535fdfdbe4b032825e56cbf8/1398792155103/PIAAC+Results+Summary+Brochure_Final_041814.pdf. Accessed March 20, 2018.

59. Centers for Disease Control and Prevention. Social media at CDC. Infographics. 2016. Available at: https://www.cdc.gov/socialmedia/tools/InfoGraphics.html. Accessed July 11, 2018.

60. Association of State and Territorial Health Officials. Available at: http://www.astho.org. Accessed March 18, 2018.

61. National Association of County & City Health Officials. Available at: http://www.naccho.org. Accessed March 20, 2018.

62. American Public Health Association. Available at: https://www.apha.org. Accessed May 3, 2018.

63. Association of Schools and Programs of Public Health. Available at: https://www.aspph.org. Accessed May 3, 2018.

64. Health Resources & Services Administration. Bureau of Primary Health Care. Available at: https://bphc.hrsa.gov. Accessed March 20, 2018.

65. US Department of Health and Human Services. SurgeonGeneral.gov. Available at: https://www.surgeongeneral.gov/index.html. Accessed March 20, 2018.

66. Centers for Disease Control and Prevention. Morbidity and mortality weekly report (MMWR). Available at: https://www.cdc.gov/mmwr/index.html. Accessed March 20, 2018.

67. Nelson DE, Hesse BW, Croyle RT. *Making Data Talk: Communicating Public Health Data to the Public, Policy Makers and the Press.* New York, NY: Oxford University Press; 2009.

68. Centers for Disease Control and Prevention. CDC health disparities & inequalities report (CHDIR). Available at: http://www.cdc.gov/minorityhealth/CHDIReport.html. Accessed March 20, 2018.

69. Centers for Disease Control and Prevention. Spina bifida. Available at: https://www.cdc.gov/ncbddd/spinabifida/toddler.html. Accessed March 20, 2018.

70. Centers for Disease Control and Prevention. Tips From Former Smokers. Available at: https://www.cdc.gov/tobacco/campaign/tips/index.html. Accessed March 20, 2018.

71. Rimal RN, Lapinski MK. Why health communication is important in public health. *Bull World Health Organ.* 2009;87:247.

3

Leadership

Donna J. Petersen, ScD, MHS, CPH

INTRODUCTION

If you search for the term "leadership" on the Internet, you will get 132 million results. On Amazon alone, you will find more than 190,000 books devoted to this subject. Strange, then, that leadership seems to be in short supply in our workplaces, in our institutions, and in our communities. Of course, this might also explain the enormous appetite for the subject. In public health, we view leadership as a critical competency for everyone working in the field, whether or not they aspire to or will ever find themselves in a "leadership" position. As such, understanding and appreciating leadership is important to the professional development of public health students, workers, and advocates. This chapter is devoted to an exploration of leadership roles and functions in public health toward promoting active leadership across the breadth and depth of the field. Some of the tasks for this topic are also covered in other chapters. In particular, this chapter will explore broad conceptualizations of leadership with the tasks associated with the leadership role in public health:

- ❑ Utilize critical analysis to prioritize and justify actions and allocation of resources.
- ❑ Apply team-building skills.
- ❑ Apply organizational change management concepts and skills.
- ❑ Apply conflict-management skills.
- ❑ Implement strategies to support and improve team performance.
- ❑ Apply negotiation skills.
- ❑ Establish and model standards of performance and accountability.
- ❑ Guide organizational decision-making and planning based on internal and external assessments.
- ❑ Prepare professional development plans for self or others.
- ❑ Develop strategies to motivate others for collaborative problem solving, decision-making, and evaluation.
- ❑ Develop capacity-building strategies at the individual, organizational, or community level.
- ❑ Communicate an organization's mission, goals, values, and shared vision to stakeholders.
- ❑ Create teams for implementing health initiatives.
- ❑ Develop a mission, goals, values, and shared vision for an organization or the community in conjunction with key stakeholders.
- ❑ Implement a continuous quality improvement plan.

❏ Develop a continuous quality improvement plan.
❏ Evaluate organizational performance in relation to strategic and defined goals.
❏ Implement organizational strategic planning processes.
❏ Assess organizational policies and procedures regarding working across multiple organizations.
❏ Align organizational policies and procedures with regulatory and statutory requirements.
❏ Maximize efficiency of programs.
❏ Ensure that informatics principles and methods are used in the design and implementation of systems.

Other Related Tasks

- Assessing needs, trends, and opportunities
- Allocating resources
- Organizational change management
- Conflict negotiation
- Team building, team performance
- Accountability
- Performance standards
- Anticipate, adapt, respond
- Continuing professional development
- Motivation for excellence
- Capacity building
- Communicating to stakeholders
- Developing vision, mission, values, goals, objectives
- Quality improvement
- Evaluation
- Policy analysis
- Promoting efficiency
- Working across agencies, sectors
- Strategic planning and strategic action

MAJOR CONTENT

Leadership Definitions

Search online for a definition of leadership and you will get more than 67 million possible responses. Here is the definition from dictionary.com:

lead·er·ship
[lee-der-ship]

noun

1. the position or function of a leader, a person who guides or directs a group:
   He managed to maintain his leadership of the party despite heavy opposition.
2. ability to lead:
   As early as sixth grade she displayed remarkable leadership potential.
3. an act or instance of leading; guidance; direction:
   They prospered under his strong leadership.
4. the leaders of a group:
   The union leadership agreed to arbitrate. [1]

Another way to clarify the meaning of a particular word is to examine the synonyms for the word. Here is a list from thesaurus.com: administration, authority, command, control, direction, influence, initiative, management, power, skill, capacity, conduction, conveyance, directorship, domination, foresight, hegemony, pilotage, preeminence, primary, superiority, and superintendency. Antonyms include impotence, inability, incapacity, powerlessness, weakness, and subservience. [2]

Leadership Theories

The interest in leadership has led to the development of numerous theories over the years about what leadership is and what makes a great leader. The "great man theory," popularized by Thomas Carlyle in the mid-1800s, supported the idea that leaders were born, not made, though critics noted that leaders were only tasked to lead because of the circumstances in which they found themselves. [3] The "trait theory," promoted by Ralph Stogdill in the 1930s, expanded on the great man theory by enumerating the personality traits that were necessary for successful leadership, though critics again noted that these did not necessarily have to be innate but could be learned depending on the leadership situation. [3]

This debate led to the development of the "behavioral theories" of the 1940s that focused more on the roles and tasks of leaders and less on intrinsic traits. These theories led to the examination of differences between leadership tasks and management tasks and led to the "contingency" theories of the 1960s that suggested that all leadership was situational. Later scholars considered "transactional" theories of leadership, which were quickly discredited and led to what we currently espouse: "transformational" theories. **Transformational theories** focus on the relationships leaders develop with others, the intrinsic personality characteristics and traits of leaders, leadership roles, and team motivation. [3]

Two leadership models that illustrate the evolution of these theories are the **McKinsey 7S Framework**[4,5] and the **Astin Social Change Model of Leadership**. [6] The McKinsey 7S Framework, developed by Thomas Peters and Robert Waterman,[4] places shared values at the center and then interconnects three hard elements (strategy, structure, and systems) and three soft elements (skills, style, and staff) to create a model for leadership within an organization or within a community.[5] The Astin model, on the other hand, identifies seven critical values, all of which begin with the letter "C": consciousness of self, congruence, commitment, collaboration, common purpose, controversy with civility, and citizenship. All of these are interconnected around the eighth "C"—*change*, which is, of course, what leadership is ultimately about.[6]

Early Development of Leadership Competencies

Most of us understand what it means to be a leader or to take a leadership role. But in public health, leadership has a specific meaning and those of us in the field have a particular responsibility to carry out the leadership that is necessary in service to the public's health. The importance of this is underscored by the fact that "leadership" was included as a core competency in the Association of Schools of Public Health's (ASPH's) first set of published competencies for the Master of Public Health (MPH) degree in 2006.[7] ASPH defined leadership as follows:

> The ability to create and communicate a shared vision for a changing future; champion solutions to organizational and community challenges; and energize commitment to goals.[7]

In that same document, a set of competencies were associated with this definition, which described the attributes of leadership in public health as follows:

- Describe alternative strategies for collaboration and partnership among organizations, focused on public health goals.
- Articulate an achievable mission, set of core values, and vision.
- Engage in dialogue and learning from others to advance public health goals.
- Demonstrate team building, negotiation, and conflict management skills.
- Demonstrate transparency, integrity, and honesty in all actions.
- Use collaborative methods for achieving organizational and community health goals.
- Apply social justice and human rights principles when addressing community needs.
- Develop strategies to motivate others for collaborative problem solving, decision-making, and evaluation.[7]

ASPH further refined the definition of leadership and the competencies associated with it when it crafted a task model for the DrPH degree, the advanced practice degree in our field, in 2009:

> The ability to create and communicate a shared vision for a positive future; inspire trust and motivate others; and use evidence-based strategies to enhance essential public health services.[8]

The following attributes of leadership extended this definition:

- "Communicate an organization's mission, shared vision, and values to stakeholders."
- "Develop teams for implementing health initiatives."

- "Collaborate with diverse groups."
- "Influence others to achieve high standards of performance and accountability."
- "Guide organizational decision-making and planning based on internal and external environmental research."
- "Prepare professional plans incorporating lifelong learning, mentoring, and continued career progression strategies."
- "Create a shared vision."
- "Develop capacity-building strategies at the individual, organizational, and community level."
- "Demonstrate a commitment to personal and professional values."[8]

Regardless of the nuances of these different explications, the gist is the same: leadership is about managing change, inspiring others, and acting within a value structure that supports improvement in the public's health, in the public's interest, and with the public's trust. This may seem like a tall order, but it is the essence of what public health practice is about. Hence, the suggestion that every public health professional must embrace his or her leadership role, regardless of organizational or societal position, gains legitimacy and importance.

Leadership in Action

Let us look at leadership as it is described in other spheres of public health. You know by now of the three core functions of public health: **assessment**, **policy development**, and **assurance**.[9] All of these functions require leadership to be carried out. These three core functions were expanded and refined in the Centers for Disease Control and Prevention's (CDC's) 10 Essential Public Health Services[10] (see Figure 3-1).

The 10 Essential Public Health Services describe the public health activities that all communities should undertake:

1. **Monitor health status** to identify and solve community health problems.
2. **Diagnose and investigate health problems and health hazards** in the community.
3. **Inform, educate, and empower** people about health issues.
4. **Mobilize community partnerships** and action to identify and solve health problems.
5. **Develop policies and plans** that support individual and community health efforts.
6. **Enforce laws and regulations** that protect health and ensure safety.
7. **Link people to needed personal health services** and assure the provision of health care when otherwise unavailable.
8. **Assure** competent public and personal health care workforce.
9. **Evaluate** effectiveness, accessibility, and quality of personal and population-based health services.
10. **Research** for new insights and innovative solutions to health problems.[11]

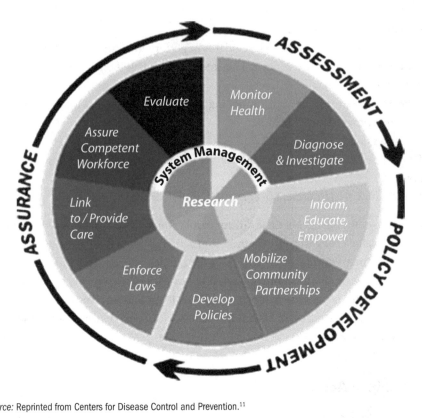

Source: Reprinted from Centers for Disease Control and Prevention.[11]

Figure 3-1. The 10 Essential Public Health Services

Again, it should be obvious that each of these tasks individually and collectively requires leadership. Indeed, these essential services form the backbone of the Public Health Accreditation Board's Standards and Measures.[12] They are used to assess the readiness of state and local public health agencies in the United States to provide quality public health services to the populations that entrust this responsibility to them. These standards also include criteria around workforce development. In that regard, three other references deserve mention.

First is the accreditation criteria promulgated by the Council on Education for Public Health for schools and programs of public health.[13] These statements about leadership are located within the required criteria. (The original numbered list was changed to a bulleted one for the purposes of this chapter.) The first statement is in regard to the MPH curriculum:

Leadership
- Apply principles of leadership, governance and management, which include creating a vision, empowering others, fostering collaboration and guiding decision making
- Apply negotiation and mediation skills to address organizational or community challenges[13]

And later in the document, for the DrPH[13]:

Leadership, Management & Governance
- Propose strategies for health improvement and elimination of health inequities by organizing stakeholders, including researchers, practitioners, community leaders and other partners
- Communicate public health science to diverse stakeholders, including individuals at all levels of health literacy, for purposes of influencing behavior and policies
- Integrate knowledge, approaches, methods, values and potential contributions from multiple professions and systems in addressing public health problems
- Create a strategic plan
- Facilitate shared decision making through negotiation and consensus-building methods
- Create organizational change strategies
- Propose strategies to promote inclusion and equity within public health programs, policies and systems
- Assess one's own strengths and weaknesses in leadership capacities, including cultural proficiency
- Propose human, fiscal and other resources to achieve a strategic goal
- Cultivate new resources and revenue streams to achieve a strategic goal[13]

Secondly, the Association of State and Territorial Health Officers completed a survey of the public health workforce in 2014,[14] which also identified several key tasks that clearly speak to a leadership role for public health professionals:

Top competency gaps and training opportunities include: policy analysis and development, business and financial management, systems thinking and social determinants of health, evidence-based public health practice, and collaborating with and engaging diverse communities.[14]

Finally, the Association of Schools and Programs of Public Health's Framing the Future Task Force, in its expert panel reports,[15] embedded leadership as part of the critical content of the core curriculum for the MPH in this way: "History and philosophy of public health as well as its core values, concepts, functions, and leadership roles"[16]; and in the critical content of the core curriculum for the DrPH, in this way: "Organizational and community leadership methods and skills, including using values clarification, developing a shared vision, conducting strategic planning, guiding decision-making, fostering collaboration, inspiring trust, and motivating others."[17] Of note, the Framing the Future Task Force was informed by a blue-ribbon panel of public health experts who noted that among the essential elements of public health education must be leadership: "Development of leadership skills to build relationships are key in order to advocate for public health and engage other parts of the health sector as well as non-health focused sectors. By inculcating elements of leadership into education, schools can ensure graduates will be prepared to lead in their chosen fields."[18]

Though not necessarily reflected in these various competency documents, one essential element of leadership is embracing the notion of professionalism (i.e., appreciating that public health is a profession in its own right, even though as a field it is comprised of skilled, committed individuals from a variety of professions and disciplines). This is a decided strength of public health but also a challenge because the field does not necessarily share the common attributes of a profession: a vocation with specialized training, a code of ethics, licensure or certification, and a commitment to lifelong learning.

Public health is a vocation, an occupation to which an individual feels particularly drawn. It also has its own specialized training leading to a terminal degree, the MPH, with baccalaureate and doctoral pathways increasingly available. It has a clearly defined code of ethics.[19] Also, it offers a certification, the Certified in Public Health (CPH), granted by the National Board of Public Health Examiners,[20] which requires maintenance of certification obtained through continuing professional development (lifelong learning). However, as not everyone comes to the field through a typical professional development pathway, it is important to at least ensure a common language and a common historical understanding of the roots of public health.

Public health is focused on populations, facilitating societies' interest in creating conditions in which everyone can be healthy. Its emphasis is on prevention, rather than treatment, and its orientation is to the community, rather than individual patients. It takes a comprehensive, holistic view incorporating models that include all aspects of the ecosystem, all the various determinants of health, a life-course perspective, and systems-level approaches. It values health equity and social justice and utilizes diverse approaches to promote overall health and well-being. While public health is ultimately a governmental responsibility (in the United States, this responsibility rests at the level of the state) many different public, private, faith-based, and nonprofit organizations contribute to public health efforts and population health improvements—hence, the need for systems-level approaches and leadership for these efforts at all levels (see Chapter 9, "Policy in Public Health," and Chapter 10, "Health Equity and Social Justice").

Levels of Leadership

So, as we have seen in this discussion, leadership in public health operates at three levels, at least. The first level is as a field: Public health has been defined as what we do collectively to create conditions in which people can be healthy.[6] This speaks to public health as a leader, championing societies' interest in enjoying good health, and doing what is necessary to realize that interest. This speaks to the notion that the field itself provides leadership in the public's interest and that, therefore, everyone working in it must embrace this leadership responsibility.

The second level is as an individual: Anyone can emerge as a leader in service to a public health cause (even when the cause is not identified as "public health" per se). Many movies and books are devoted to the notion of the hero-leader who singlehandedly takes on a challenge, fights whatever institution is in the way, and wins the good fight. Many of these are in health-related areas (e.g., *Silkwood* [1983], *Contagion* [2011]). Everyday people engage in similarly courageous work, whether it be around school bus safety or genetically modified organism (GMO) labeling of foods. This type of local advocacy requires a leader or leaders to emerge to maintain the momentum needed to address the issue. This level also includes public health professionals or persons in related organizations who accept responsibility for a particular task and provide the leadership necessary to see it through.

The third level is what we more typically think of when we talk about leadership and that is the roles and responsibilities of the person or persons in leadership positions. Let us pause for a moment and think about *leaders* in public health—do any come to mind? Students often suggest Reverend Dr. Martin Luther King Jr. or President Barack Obama. If they are old enough to remember, they may suggest Surgeon General Dr. C. Everett Koop. What do these men have in common? They were visionaries, they inspired others, they took risks to achieve what they believed to be important goals, and they motivated others to be bold in tackling pressing social problems. These are key attributes of leaders and these translate from the highest offices to a work team or even to a neighborhood. You do not have to be at the top of the organization chart to practice good leadership. Other key attributes of leadership include honesty, integrity, humility, and empathy. Good leaders are good communicators: They listen well and are open to new ideas. They motivate, delegate, congratulate, share credit, and champion their colleagues. They are good partners, capable of building coalitions, and are experts at resolving conflicts.

Are leaders born? Some are, certainly. But they can also be made, by learning the underlying behaviors that lead to success and avoiding those tactics that demoralize a team and stifle creative, committed action.

Because leadership is a popular topic, many tools have been developed to help individuals understand their leadership styles, strengths, and areas for improvement. Instruments such as the Myers-Briggs Type Indicator[21] and the DiSC[22] profile provide a window into an individual's preferences for communicating, collaborating, or thriving in a work environment. If you have not yet had an opportunity to complete one of these instruments, it is worth doing, particularly in a facilitated setting. Gaining insights into your own attributes and the things that trigger your less desirable traits can be a helpful start on the path to learning good leadership techniques and methods.

One of leadership's great challenges is that the leader often finds himself or herself also serving as a manager. There is an important distinction between these two roles, most easily summarized in the following idea attributed to Warren Bennis: "Leaders do the right things, managers do things right."[23] The manager of a production line does not need to think creatively; he or she just needs to make sure everything happens as it should with maximum efficiency and productivity. Managers are typically internally focused. Leaders, on the other hand, need to be externally focused, watching for trends, interacting with decision-makers and power-brokers, considering new product lines, or anticipating changes in the industry. When one person is asked to do both tasks, one usually gets short shrift; the literature would suggest that it is the leadership function that typically suffers.

Leadership is essential in public health as it is necessary to always be scanning the horizon and anticipating changes that may have an impact on the public's health. Leadership is essential to articulating the bold vision of public health: **health is a human right** and everyone deserves the opportunity to grow and live in health. Leadership is also essential to translate that vision into a mission and a set of goals and objectives that can be communicated, shared, modified, and ultimately embraced toward collective effort. Leadership is essential in developing plans that can be articulated, evaluated, and discussed with all constituency groups. Leadership is essential in communicating a shared vision for the change that is always necessary to continually promote population health.

PRACTICE QUESTIONS

See if you understand leadership decisions by reading through the following examples of leadership in action and putting yourself in the leader position:

1. A state health officer learns of an outbreak of meningitis in a small, but densely populated community that includes a college. Available data suggest that this population has not been vaccinated against this disease and the literature indicates that the disease can be fatal or result in serious permanent disability. It is near the end of the fiscal year, so scant resources are available. On the advice of her epidemiologists and medical staff, the state health officer orders the purchase of sufficient vaccine to create herd immunity in the population; develops a priority list for vaccination; deploys all available personnel to administer the vaccine in the town; directs her communications department to notify community leaders, the media, and the general public of the outbreak and the steps being taken to control it; and notifies the governor and key members of the legislature of her decision. The crisis is averted, but she then has to advocate with the legislature for an emergency appropriation to cover the costs of this response. She also approaches the health insurance companies that dominate the market in the community to ask for their financial support. A compromise is reached; all is well.

2. Late on a Friday, a local health department staff person is finishing up some paperwork when a frantic man runs in the door to say his wife is in labor. They were turned away from the local hospital for being uninsured and they have run out of gas. The staff person, alone in the office, has a cash box in the drawer in front of her but nowhere in the rules does it say it can be used for a purpose like this. Looking again at the stricken man and wanting to help she thinks about her options and the risk she is running if she chooses incorrectly; her job could be on the line as well as that of her boss. Casting those fears aside, she gives the man money out of the cashbox for gas, tells him to bring his wife inside, and gets on the phone. Eventually, she finds a nurse-midwife who agrees to come to the health department to assess the woman and her level of risk and an obstetrician who is willing to be on the phone to help triage. She keeps calling hospitals until she finds one who is willing to take them, but when the nurse-midwife arrives, it is too late to transport the mother. Enlisting the help of the staff person and with the doctor on the phone, they successfully deliver the baby. Dad gets back with the gas in time to take both to the hospital awaiting their arrival. Monday morning, the staff person did not lose her job; instead, she was given a hero's welcome.

3. A well-to-do community that is supportive of clean energy agrees to have wind energy turbines located near their residences. Almost immediately after the turbines are installed and operational, the residents begin experiencing negative health effects. Forming a coalition, the residents seek to confirm that their health effects are related to the turbines by inviting experts to help them assess the situation. After trying every avenue, they reluctantly petition the county to have them removed or relocated. After several years and much legal wrangling, a judge sides with them declaring the turbines a nuisance. They are shut down pending an appeal from the county. In the meantime, the residents are having their health carefully monitored to determine if there might have been some other cause for their problems. Though the community supports clean energy, the county decides not to file an appeal and the turbines are permanently shut down.

These all exemplify leadership in action, whether undertaken by a leader, a staff member, or a community. They also reflect some of the other tasks of leaders, as identified in the Job Task Analysis conducted in 2014 by the National Board of Public Health Examiners.[20] This survey was completed by more than 4,000 people who identified themselves as working in public health and identified the most critical tasks essential to their work. It is proficiency at these tasks that the CPH examination tests.[24]

LEADERSHIP TASKS IN NATURAL CLUSTERS

Let us consider these tasks in some natural clusters. The first includes those tasks related to the core public health function of **assessment**.[9] Leaders are always scanning the horizon, monitoring available data, and engaging in dialogue with other community leaders and stakeholders to identify trends, consider changing circumstances, and anticipate needs. From the information they collect, leaders ensure that they design and implement data systems with integrity to meet the identified needs while respecting privacy concerns of individuals. Informatics principles are applied to accomplish this. Leaders are also always on the lookout for opportunities to engage new partners, address new or persistent challenges, or modify approaches to health challenges.

In the spirit of an inclusive approach to public health, leaders also engage in regular dialogue with leaders from other sectors, elected officials, and the general public. They do this to continually keep abreast of emerging challenges or opportunities for community health promotion. Though leaders respect the importance of a strategic, data-informed, and community-engaged planning process, they are also highly attuned to changing circumstances, anticipating, adapting, and responding to community health needs.

Assessment is also dependent on high-quality monitoring and **evaluation**, not only to ensure that programs and interventions are addressing the needs identified in productive ways, but also to promote **accountability** for the public's trust and public funds. Good leaders recognize that they must also be good stewards of the public's trust and the public funds provided to them, and that they must use their funds and their leadership skills to promote health and safety and to prevent disease and the negative consequences of disease and injury.

Leaders value data of all kinds, quantitative and qualitative, and accept the responsibility of balancing the natural political nature of their work with as much evidence as possible in order to make informed decisions. Public health agencies collect, access, and utilize vast amounts of data on the populations they serve and accept the accountability and confidentiality rules that govern such use. They also respect the importance of data-based decision-making, including in the performance evaluations of their agencies, programs, and staff. Good leaders embrace **performance standards** for their agencies, their programs, and their staff, and ensure that evaluations at all levels are conducted routinely and feedback offered constructively. They are knowledgeable about and regularly employ **quality improvement** strategies and they are comfortable communicating the results of evaluations and assessments with stakeholders, including policymakers, the media, clients, and the general public.

The second set of tasks includes those relating to **management**. As we noted earlier, few leaders have the luxury of not also serving as managers though they typically oversee a group of high-level managers who are responsible for specific programmatic efforts. One important management task performed by leaders is the **allocation of resources** to accomplish agency or program goals and objectives. The creation of a **strategic plan** related to a clearly stated **vision** and **mission statement** for the agency is also an important task in program management; the overarching structure of such a plan informs the selection and measurement of relevant goals and measurable objectives. The leader is also the keeper of the **values** of the organization, articulating them clearly to both employees and the public, holding professionals accountable to them and linking all elements of the strategic plan back to them.

In addition to effectively communicating such plans, goals, and strategies to staff, other agencies, and the general public, leaders also commit to **capacity building** in all sectors relevant to the public health work of the agency. This can include **continuing professional development** of staff and partners, effectively communicating with and engaging stakeholders, and working to eliminate barriers to the efficient deployment of public health resources and strategies. In this regard, public health leaders have to be adept at working across sectors, agencies, institutions, and communities to promote understanding of public health challenges, seek ideas for and consensus around strategies to address them, and motivate action toward solutions.

As public health is often accomplished through analysis, development, and enactment of policy strategies, public health leaders must also be adept at managing the **policymaking process**. Former Surgeon General Julius B. Richmond and his colleague Milton Kotelchuck, in a model they developed,[25,26] posit that leaders must cultivate within the community an understanding of the problem being addressed, consensus around the appropriate solution, and the political will to act on what is often an unpopular solution.

The third set of tasks thus revolves around **managing change**, both within the organization being led and the community being served. Because as societies we do not often agree on the nature of the problems facing us and certainly not on possible solutions (consider climate change in the United States in the 2000s), public health efforts invite dissent and thus require leaders to be excellent at **managing conflict** and at **negotiating**. Entire books have been written on these subjects as well (e.g., *Crucial Conversations: Tools for Talking When Stakes Are High* by Patterson et al.[27]). Any are worth a read as there is always more to be learned on these critical subjects. As challenging as these tasks are in a highly charged political environment—which governmental public health is—it is also challenging to manage change within an organization.

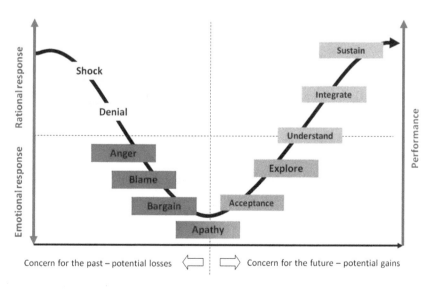

Source: Reprinted with permission from Green.[28]

Figure 3-2. The Human Response to Change Cycle

It is a strangely typical characteristic of humans that we prefer the familiar and are uncomfortable with change. Think about encountering a road closure on your way home from work. For most of us, a "detour" sign not only generates feelings of annoyance but also often feelings of fear. Similarly, being moved to a new office, being assigned to a new supervisor, or being pulled off one project and placed on another generates similar feelings of annoyance and, yes, of fear. Leaders understand this and utilize tools available to manage organizational change. Consider Figure 3-2, which represents the human response to change: what it suggests is that change management is just that—change has to be managed.

Leaders respect that people have to work through all the stages of change in order to adapt and emerge stronger and more productive. In public health, great leaders recognize that this is not just true of employees, but also true of the public, especially those who utilize public health services and are similarly change-averse.

CONCLUSION

In summary, leadership is a necessary ingredient for public health success that is often in short supply. Whether within organizations, teams, or the community at large, embracing the important role of leadership and utilizing effective leadership tools can make an enormous difference in whether and how public health goals are achieved. As a public health professional, it is in your best interest to understand this important function/service/competency/job task and master its principles. Living the values of public health, accepting responsibility for the task at hand, and practicing with honesty, integrity, and humility will facilitate your path to leadership in public health.

REFERENCES

1. Leadership. Dictionary.com. Available at: http://www.dictionary.com/browse/leadership. Accessed July 7, 2017.

2. Leadership. *Roget's 21st Century Thesaurus*. 3rd ed. Available at: http://www.thesaurus.com/browse/leadership. Accessed July 7, 2017.

3. Leadership theories. Leadership-central.com. Available at: http://www.leadership-central.com/leadership-theories.html#axzz4oysDbIEs. Accessed August 6, 2017.

4. Peters TJ, Waterman RH. *In Search of Excellence: Lessons from America's Best-Run Companies.* 1st ed. New York, NY: Harper & Row; 1982.

5. Lowell B. Enduring ideas: The 7-S framework. *McKinsey Quarterly*. March 2008. Available at: https://www.mckinsey.com/business-functions/strategy-and-corporate-finance/our-insights/enduring-ideas-the-7-s-framework. Accessed August 6, 2017.

6. Astin HS. Leadership for social change. *About Campus*. 1996;1(3):4–10.

7. ASPPH Masters in Public Health Degree Core Competency Model Version 2.3. Washington, DC: Association of Schools and Programs of Public Health; 2006.

8. ASPPH Doctor of Public Health (DrPH) Core Competency Model Version 1.3. Washington, DC: Association of Schools and Programs of Public Health; 2009.

9. Institute of Medicine. *The Future of Public Health*. Washington, DC: The National Academies Press; 1988.

10. Centers for Disease Control and Prevention. National Public Health Performance Standards. 2017. Available at: https://www.cdc.gov/nphpsp/essentialservices.html. Accessed July 7, 2017.

11. Centers for Disease Control and Prevention. The public health system & the 10 Essential Public Health Services. Available at: https://www.cdc.gov/stltpublichealth/publichealthservices/essentialhealthservices.html. Accessed June 23, 2018.

12. Public Health Accreditation Board. Public Health Accreditation Board Standards & Measures, version 1.5. Available at: http://www.phaboard.org/wp-content/uploads/PHABSM_WEB_LR1.pdf. Accessed July 7, 2017.

13. Council on Education for Public Health. Accreditation criteria: schools of public health and public health programs. 2016. Available at: https://storage.googleapis.com/media.ceph.org/wp_assets/2016.Criteria.pdf.. Accessed July 7, 2017.

14. Association of State and Territorial Health Officials. 2014 public health workforce interests and needs survey (PH WINS). Available at: http://www.astho.org/phwins. Accessed August 4, 2017.

15. Association of Schools and Programs of Public Health. Framing the future. 2015. Available at: https://www.aspph.org/teach-research/framing-the-future. Accessed July 7, 2017.

16. Association of Schools and Programs of Public Health. The MPH degree: transition to a 21st century model. 2015. Available at: https://www.aspph.org/ftf-reports/the-mph. Accessed July 7, 2017.

17. Association of Schools and Programs of Public Health. The DrPH degree prepares transformative leaders. 2015. Available at: https://www.aspph.org/ftf-reports/the-drph. Accessed July 7, 2017.

18. Association of Schools and Programs of Public Health. Blue ribbon employers advisory board report: trends in public health education. Available at: https://www.aspph.org/ftf-reports/blue-ribbon-employer-advisory-board-report. Accessed July 7, 2017.

19. Public Health Leadership Society. Principles of the ethical practice of public health. 2002. Available at: https://www.apha.org/-/media/files/pdf/membergroups/ethics/ethics_brochure.ashx?la=en&hash=1E9425A9C96347E42AC0D6B0D2000AA6A8717C3C. Accessed June 13, 2018.

20. National Board of Public Health Examiners. CPH certified in public health. Available at: https://www.nbphe.org. Accessed August 4, 2017.

21. The Myers & Briggs Foundation. MBTI basics. Available at: https://www.myersbriggs.org/my-mbti-personality-type/mbti-basics/home.htm?bhcp=1. Accessed June 14, 2018.

22. Wiley. Everything DiSC. Available at: https://www.wiley.com/WileyCDA/Brand/id-43.html. Accessed August 4, 2017.

23. Bennis WG, Nanus B. *Leaders: The Strategies for Taking Charge.* New York, NY: HarperPerennial; 1985.

24. National Board of Public Health Examiners. Job task analysis survey. Available at: https://www.nbphe.org/job-task-analysis. Accessed August 8, 2017.

25. Atwood K, Colditz GA, Kawachi I. From public health science to prevention policy: placing science in its social and political contexts. *Am J Public Health.* 1997;87(10):1603–1606.

26. Richmond JB, Kotelchuck M. Coordination and development of strategies and policy for public health promotion in the US. In: *Oxford Textbook of Public Health.* 2nd ed. London, England: Oxford University Press; 1991:441–454.

27. Patterson K, Grenny J, McMillan R, Switzler A, Roppe L. *Crucial Conversation: Tools for Talking When the Stakes Are High.* New York, NY: McGraw-Hill; 2002.

28. Green S. Managing change in the workplace. Love-Monday-Mornings. Available at: http://www.love-monday-mornings.com/managing-change-work-place. Accessed June 23, 2018.

4

Law and Ethics

Katherine Drabiak, JD, and Zachary Pruitt, PhD, MHA, CPH

INTRODUCTION

Public health law and ethics provide the framework for decision-making regarding interventions that keep populations healthy. Public health laws are the formal practices enforced by authorities exemplified by statutes, regulations, and court decisions. Public health ethics arise from informal policies and codes of professional conduct to guide public health practice. Competent public health professionals understand the basics of public health law and its application to ethical research and practice.

Public health laws address the government's power and duty to protect the public's health and the limitations on those powers.[1] Public health practitioners frequently encounter situations in which the promotion of community health conflicts with individual rights. The practice of public health law balances assurance of the common good with the protection of civil liberties.

Ethics play an important complementary role to public health law. The term "public health ethics" refers to the discipline that examines what practices make good conduct in a particular situation or dilemma.[2] The study of ethics helps public health practitioners determine and justify the most appropriate course of action.

By the end of this chapter, you should be able to apply the following tasks:

☐ Identify regulations regarding health privacy, security, confidentiality (e.g., personal health information).

☐ Design strategies to ensure implementation of laws and regulations governing the scope of one's legal authority.

☐ Apply basic principles of ethical analysis to issues of public health research, practice, and policy.

☐ Ensure the application of ethical principles in the collection, maintenance, use, and dissemination of data and information.

☐ Manage potential conflicts of interest encountered by practitioners, researchers, and organizations.

☐ Advise on the laws, regulations, policies, and procedures for the ethical conduct of public health research, practice, and policy.

❑ Identify environmental, social justice, and other factors that contribute to health disparities.

❑ Apply social justice and human rights principles when addressing community needs.

MAJOR CONTENT

Public Health Law

Government has the power and duty to enforce public health laws, but the authority is limited.[1] To explain this tension more fully, this section will first explain the legal basis for the US federal government's public health powers to protect community health. Next, it will evaluate how the roles of the different parts of government serve the public's health through laws and regulations. This section will also describe how laws and regulations relate to each other by using health privacy, security, and confidentiality examples. Finally, it will describe the federal, state, and local governments' authority to enforce public health laws and how these powers can be limited to protect individual freedoms.

Federal Public Health Powers

The US Constitution is one of many sources of law but is considered the "supreme Law of the Land."[3] Although the Constitution does not specifically refer to public health, it gives certain powers to the federal government to protect community health. These federal powers include the power to regulate interstate commerce in the Commerce Clause (i.e., laws concerning goods sold across state lines), the power to tax and spend (e.g., taxing tobacco products and federal grants on health programs), and the Necessary and Proper Clause (i.e., when Congress makes a law to help carry out one of its listed powers).[1] Under the Supremacy Clause in the US Constitution, if there is a difference between federal law and state law or interpretation, the federal law will prevail.

The relationship of the federal government to the state governments is expressly established in the US Constitution. **Federalism** is the term that describes the distribution of power between the individual states and national government.[1] Under federalism, the Constitution expressly establishes areas in which the federal government, through Congress, can enact laws, including those pertaining to public health. In areas where the federal government seeks a uniform approach or policy, Congress may pass federal legislation for the state to adopt. For example, consider state minimum drinking age laws. If one state had lower minimum drinking age laws than another, this may encourage traveling across state lines to drink, traveling back to one's home state, and increasing intoxicated drivers on interstate roadways.[4] Here, the federal government has an interest in reducing drunk drivers. Congress enacted a law that made states adopt the federal standard for minimum drinking age a condition for receiving federal highway construction funds.[5]

***

Vignette 1: *The Patient Protection and Affordable Care Act of 2010 (ACA) required most legal US citizens to purchase health insurance. Linda, an employee of the State Department of Health, knew that the governor of her state opposed the passage of the federal legislation. Linda's boss asked her to write a memo to the health department staff that explained why the people of the state would be required to comply with the mandate that individuals buy health insurance.*

What legal issue should Linda address in the memo?

On the basis of the principles of federalism, Linda should explain that citizens of her state would be required to purchase health insurance even though the governor of the state disagrees with the federal law. The Supreme Court upheld the individual mandate of the ACA, finding that Congress was within the bounds of its authority to enact legislation requiring individuals to purchase health insurance.[6]

***

Relationship Between Laws and Regulations

Both the state and federal levels of government contain three branches: the Legislative Branch, the Executive Branch, and the Judicial Branch. The Legislative Branch makes law, the Executive Branch implements the law, and the Judicial Branch interprets the law. Your understanding of the relationship among the different branches of government is critical to effective public health practice.

Public health **laws** are the system of rules created for the protection or promotion of community health.[1] **Regulations** are the set of rules that describe the implementation of legislation.[1] Both legislation and regulation are similar in that they carry the force of law, but different in that legislation is produced by the legislative branch (i.e., Congress) and regulation is promulgated through the executive branch (i.e., the president and administrative agencies, such as the Centers for Disease Control and Prevention or the Food and Drug Administration).[2]

Once Congress passes a law that requires regulations, the administrative agency of the Executive Branch must stay within the bounds of the authority granted by Congress and follow specific procedures for **rulemaking** set forth in federal law. First, the administrative agency issues a notice of proposed rulemaking. Then, the regulatory agency will publish a Notice of Proposed Rulemaking (a draft) in the *Federal Register,* which explains the issue and how the agency plans to address it. During this time, interested parties and stakeholders may draft comments and provide feedback on important issues to consider. The administrative agency may consider these comments but has discretion as to whether and how it takes them into consideration when drafting the Final Rule. The Final Rule is then published in the Code of Federal Regulations and has the force of law. A similar rulemaking process also happens at the state level.

One example of how legislation and regulation work in tandem can be seen in a 1996 federal law called the **Health Insurance Portability and Accountability Act (HIPAA)**. HIPAA governs patient rights pertaining to the uses, disclosure, and access to individual health information.[7,8] HIPAA attempts to balance the inappropriate sharing of identifiable health information while promoting the flow of health information for health care and public health uses.[7,8] Congress passed HIPAA and then the Department of Health and Human Services, through the Office of Civil Rights, created regulations to implement the law.

The HIPAA regulations are known as the HIPAA Privacy Rule and the HIPAA Security Rule.[7,8] Both regulations define the rules for use, disclosure, and protection of protected health information. **Protected health information (PHI)** is any identifiable information about an individual including demographic data, physical or mental health condition, or receipt of health care services.[1] HIPAA rules apply to certain entities referred to as **covered entities**, such as health care providers, health care plans, and health care clearinghouses.[1] There is no restriction on the use or disclosure of de-identified health information.[1]

Privacy refers to the freedom from intrusion and having control over the extent, timing, and circumstances of sharing one's information.[9] The HIPAA Privacy Rule specifies circumstances in which a covered entity may use and disclose PHI, including when an individual's authorization is required for the entity to share the PHI. For example, an entity may share the medical records of a patient without the patient's authorization under the normal operation of health services delivery, including treatment, coordination of care, or payment. **Security** is defined as the practices, policies, and procedures created to protect a person's PHI.[1] The HIPAA Security Rule defines appropriate organizational and technological safeguards (e.g., passwords, encryption) to protect the privacy of PHI.

The HIPAA Privacy Rule contains additional **permitted disclosures** relating to public safety and welfare,[10] such as disclosing PHI of victims of abuse to appropriate authorities. State-based agencies that investigate and advocate for those who cannot care for themselves or need assistance, such as children and the elderly, are an example of *parens patriae*. *Parens patriae* refers to state legal action on behalf of individuals who cannot protect themselves, such as suspected victims of child neglect or elder abuse.[1] The HIPAA Privacy Rule also permits disclosures to law enforcement for certain types of wounds or physical injuries, such as gunshot wounds.[11]

***

Vignette 2: *Mildred, a nurse at the County Hospital, overhears a conversation between Dr. Grey and a patient. The patient seeks treatment for his sexually transmitted disease. Mildred takes a photo of the patient and publicly posts it to social media, with the County Hospital logo in the background and the caption "Public service message: steer clear of this charmer. Just treated for an STD."*

Which HIPAA rule pertains to this vignette?

Mildred's post to social media constitutes a **breach** of the HIPAA Privacy Rule, in which an entity or individual discloses PHI without an individual authorization that does not fall under a listed exception or permitted uses.[1] Here, Mildred breached the Privacy Rule because she disclosed the identity of the patient through his photo, disclosed his medical condition, and disclosed the fact he received treatment at the County Hospital. Both federal law and state law specify penalties for accidental (e.g., laptop with patient information stolen from a car) and intentional (e.g., illegally selling patient information) breaches.

In Vignette 2, Dr. Grey also has a duty of confidentiality in relation to the patient. **Confidentiality** refers to the patient disclosing information in a relationship of trust with Dr. Grey and the patient's expectation that Dr. Grey will not inappropriately divulge this information to others without permission.[1] Confidentiality can be expressly promised or factually implied, such as in the physician–patient relationship. State medical licensing statutes and professional regulations have a duty of confidentiality.[1] An exception to confidentiality is made for mandatory reporting of infectious disease to or by public health agencies.[1] **Public health surveillance** refers to the "acquisition, use, retention, and transmission of data about the population's health that supports essential functions of the public health system."[1] In Vignette 2, the **public health exception** permits Dr. Grey to report the patient's PHI to the state health department for the limited purpose of STD surveillance.[12]

***

Vignette 3: *A state-based prescription drug monitoring program tracks opioid prescriptions and collects from pharmacies certain identifiable patient data, including name, address, date of birth, and sex. To curb the rising opioid addiction affecting the citizens of her state, the Commissioner of Health proposes that health department staff access the prescription drug monitoring program and analyze the database to proactively identify potential abusers. If the health department staff identifies a pattern of unnecessary opioid use, then the health department staff would notify law enforcement authorities to investigate.*

What issues does the Commissioner's proposal raise?

HIPAA regulations *permit* state laws to specify situations in which health practitioners are *required* to report conditions to appropriate state agencies, called **mandatory**

reporting.[1] However, the Commissioner's proposal illustrates the limitations on reporting of PHI. Principles of **confidentiality** are violated if PHI is shared with law enforcement beyond the original scope of prescription drug monitoring programs described in Vignette 3. Most prescription drug databases are intended to provide a resource for clinicians to assess whether a patient has been prescribed other medications. They are not intended as a tool to gather information for law enforcement purposes. Many state health departments use de-identified records in the prescription drug monitoring database to track the impact of the prescription drug monitoring program on general rates of opioid use in the state.

The Commissioner's proposal would also violate the **Fourth Amendment** of the US Constitution's protection against unreasonable search and seizure.[1] Many programs collect health information under the authority of the state for purposes, such as surveillance and monitoring.[1] In general, however, law enforcement may not obtain (search or seize) the information contained in such databases without a warrant and probable cause.[9]

***

Scope of Authority and Limitations of Government Power

In the US Constitution, the **10th Amendment** enables states to exercise all powers that are neither given to the federal government nor prohibited by the Constitution.[1] States may pass laws designed to promote the health, safety, and welfare of its residents under the authority of police power. **Police powers** are the coercive powers of states to enact laws and promulgate regulations to protect the public and to promote the common good.[1] Note that the state is involved in the application of police power, not the federal government. The federal government is not allowed to use police power, so states retain police powers designed to protect the public's health. Examples of public health police powers include isolation of a man with tuberculosis (a limitation on his liberty) or destroying barrels of contaminated poultry from a distributor (destruction of their property).[1]

At times, individuals or groups may object to state laws that use police power because the law impinges on their **autonomy**, to be free from external influence over independent decision-making.[1] Laws may either compel action or constrain action, which can be seen in the context of communicable disease and vaccination laws.

***

Vignette 4: *A state law where Sally lives requires vaccination for all children entering the public school system. Sally objects to vaccination for her child because of fears that vaccines can create other health risks. Sally also points out that the school has a policy that requires sick children to remain at home until the child is no longer contagious.*

What public health law concept allows the state to require Sally's child to be vaccinated as a condition of entering the public school system?

In the seminal case, *Jacobson v. Massachusetts* in 1905, the Supreme Court upheld a state law in Massachusetts that required either compulsory vaccination of adult residents against smallpox or required the individual to pay a fine as a proper exercise of the state's **police power**.[13] The court found that states, through local health authorities, may exercise its police power to impose reasonable regulations pertaining to **mandatory vaccination** to protect the public against the imminent danger of a threatened epidemic of communicable disease.[13] Since *Jacobson v. Massachusetts*, states have enacted specific laws tying vaccination mandates to school attendance because states view this as an effective measure to protect the public from communicable disease, specifically when children are gathered in close quarters such as school.[14]

***

The state may also enact laws or regulations that constrain individual action or place conditions on individual liberty if the state determines that these conditions are essential to the safety, peace, health, and order of the community.[1] This may include measures to separate individuals or constrain their movement to prevent the spread of communicable disease. **Isolation** is the separation of an infected person for the time period that they could transmit a contagious disease to other people.[1] **Quarantine** is the detention of healthy persons who may have been exposed to contagious disease during the period of incubation to prevent transmission of infections.[1] In addition to *state*-based public health authority, the Public Health Service Act delegated authority to the Centers for Disease Control and Prevention to intervene on the *federal level* to detain, isolate, or quarantine to control the spread of communicable disease between the states or into the country.[15]

In some cases, the individual may not wish to comply with isolation or related treatment measures.[9] In that instance, the state may seek a **civil commitment order**, which confines an individual in a medical facility for a specific period of treatment.[16] The state would need to show that the individual has a communicable disease and poses a risk of injury to others. Civil commitment generally refers to when an individual indicates intent not to comply with treatment. Civil commitment hearings by a court also require **due process**, in which the individual must be given notice of the hearing, be offered an opportunity to object, and be permitted to present his own evidence before a court can decide whether to deprive the individual of liberty.[9] Even then, public health practitioners should achieve community health in a way that respects the rights of individuals in the community by asking whether any **less restrictive alternatives** of treatment are possible.[9]

Public health authorities have a variety of tools to enforce public health laws and regulations, including inspections, licensing, and nuisance abatement.[1] Courts have ruled that inspections of dangerous and commonly regulated industries without warrants are allowed under certain limitations.[1] When conducting inspections of businesses, public health authorities seek needed information in order to implement effective policies that protect community health.

Public health authorities may also use public nuisance law to take steps to control an activity or prohibit an activity that poses a public health threat. **Nuisance abatement** is the control of the interference with a community's use of public space or the public's common welfare, such as improper sewage disposal or use of explosives.[1]

***

Vignette 5: *Jerry is an inspector for the division of chemical laboratory for the state department of health. He presented his credentials to the president of AgriChem stating his authority to conduct a surprise inspection and review of license for the chemical manufacturing facility. The president of AgriChem refused to allow Jerry to inspect the facility stating that it was a warrantless inspection.*

Under what legal authority can Jerry inspect the manufacturing facility?

In Vignette 5, Jerry is acting on behalf of the state department of health, which has the authority to conduct inspections to protect public health. Many businesses or professions must be permitted or **licensed** by the state, county, or local health department to operate.[1] Although the **Fourth Amendment** to the Constitution protects against unreasonable searches and seizures, licensed businesses, such as food producers and chemical manufacturers, are subject to warrantless random inspections to enforce safety standards.[1] In instances in which permits or licenses are not required, administrative warrants can be obtained through the courts in order to protect the public's health.[1]

***

Public Health Ethics

According to the Centers for Disease Control and Prevention,[2] public health ethics refers to our inquiry or examination about what is good conduct and about our decision-making process when confronted with dilemmas about what is the right course of action. Furthermore, ethical judgments must be made within the relevant social context that may change over time. Public health ethical practice also recognizes that for certain complex issues there is no right answer. There may be a good and sound answer that is perhaps preferred among other alternatives, but it may still be laden with problems and criticisms.

This section will first explain how public health professionals can apply human rights, environmental justice, and social justice principles when addressing community needs. Next, it will describe basic principles of ethical analysis of public health research, practice, and policy issues using a three-step framework to decision-making. This section will also examine the fundamental ethical concepts and theories to issues of public health research, practice, and policy.

Human Rights and Social Justice

The foundation of public health ethics recognizes a right to health and basic human rights. International treaties, such as the Universal Declaration of Human Rights drafted by the United Nations sets forth **human rights principles**, such as freedom, equality, equal protection under the law, and "the right to a standard of living adequate for the health and well-being of himself and his family."[17] The American Public Health Association Code of Ethics[18] has affirmed the right to health as a general ethical principle. As a related concept, the **egalitarian** principle says that public health interventions should ensure equal protection according to the notion that all people are equal.[19]

***

Vignette 6: *Hubert, a homeless man, presents in the local health department's community clinic with active tuberculosis. Hubert explains to the nurse that he has been staying at Community Services, a local homeless shelter. He is willing to comply with the medical team's recommendations for tuberculosis treatment. Hubert's diagnosis is a part of an increase of active tuberculosis cases among the homeless population in the area.*

Under what ethical principal should health department officials plan to investigate the living conditions of the local homeless population in order to decrease the amount of active tuberculosis cases?

Vignette 6 raises the ethical concept of social justice. **Social justice** refers to what is "fair, equitable, and appropriate treatment in light of what is due or owed groups."[1] Social justice requires that public health practitioners examine questions of how some groups face disproportionate risk of disease, called **health disparities**.[20] Socially disadvantaged populations, such as the homeless or those living in poverty, are at increased risk of disease, including active tuberculosis infection.[20] Public health practice should examine the **fundamental causes** of disease, such as environmental conditions, occupational exposures, genetics, or lifestyle factors.[18] In Vignette 6, public health interventions could address the close living quarters at the homeless shelter, lack of sanitary resources associated with homelessness, or other preventable factors that may compromise immune function among the homeless.[9]

Now, using the facts in Vignette 6, if County Hospital experienced a medication shortage and did not have sufficient medication to treat all patients presenting with tuberculosis, then this would raise the concern of distributive justice. **Distributive justice** refers to the just allocation of benefits.[19] In Vignette 6, distributive justice would refer to the fair allocation of medication among persons who are ill and not allocating less resources to disfavored groups, such as the poor and homeless.

***

Vignette 7: *One morning, 12 patients present in the emergency department at County Hospital with the same symptoms of nausea, headache, vomiting, and convulsions. One of the patients, Carlos, is able to tell the physician that he and the rest of the patients are farmworkers. As they were working on Berry Farm this morning, an airplane flew overhead spraying the fields and workers with pesticides. Carlos tells the physician that most of the farmworkers on Berry Farm are recent immigrants from Mexico, and their job provides the best opportunity to economically provide for their families. Health Advocates, a nonprofit organization, begins a project examining different rates of exposure to pesticides between immigrant farmworkers versus the general public.*

Which concept would be most relevant if Health Advocates plans to use this information to lobby for pesticide regulatory reform?

Carlos indicated that farm work was one of the best options to provide for his family, yet this exposed him to acute health hazards associated with pesticide contact. This example raises the concept of environmental justice. **Environmental justice** means the fair treatment of all people in the application of public health policy that reduces disparity in the exposure to environmental contamination.[9] **Health disparities** often *result* from environmental injustice.[19] In Vignette 7, health disparities would refer to differences in the population of farmworkers suffering higher incidence of disease arising from pesticide exposure, as compared with other population groups.

***

Steps in Ethical Decision-Making

In professions, codes of ethics establish the rules for professional behavior. The Code of Ethics for Public Health is a list of moral norms of public health practitioners that can be used as a guide for addressing the increasingly complex ethical dilemmas in day-to-day practice.[18] The public health ethics framework is not a simple formula, but rather is a series of questions designed to provoke rigorous deliberation among public health professionals. The steps to ethical decision-making may include (1) analyzing the ethical issues, (2) evaluating the ethical dimensions of the various public health options, and (3) providing justification for one particular public health action.[21]

***

Vignette 8: *The water detention basins that protect the community of Agresta Ranch from flooding when water does not drain properly are not working as they should. To prevent the spread of mosquito-borne disease in the suburban community, the local health department plans to cite the residents for violation of the nuisance law that protects the community from stagnant water. Jerry, a new health department employee, proposes that the health department repair the detention basins at no charge to the community. In return, the community would agree to let Jerry conduct a mosquito breeding study at Agresta Ranch that compares the mosquito breeding rates of newly repaired detention basins versus the detention basins with stagnant water.*

As Jerry's boss, you need to analyze the ethical issues associated with his proposal. Which is the most important ethical concept you should consider in your deliberation in this situation?

    a. Legal authority
    b. Informed consent
    c. Stakeholder input
    d. Risk analysis

Answer: d. Risk analysis, and let us explore why.

As a preliminary note, health departments have the **legal authority** under state nuisance laws to penalize residents for stagnant water in detention basins because of the potential health risks associated with mosquito-borne disease. The law also permits health officials to conduct certain types of public health research.

Next, health officials may consider whether community consent to an intervention is required. The American Public Health Association Code of Ethics[18] requires public health institutions to obtain the community's **informed consent** for interventions, and the vignette states that the "community would agree." Presumably, any agreement with the community to conduct research in exchange for repairing the detention basins would include informed consent forms. However, it could be argued that, even with informed consent in this scenario, the research proposal would be unethical because of the pressure that residents of Agresta Ranch would feel to avoid the citations for the stagnant water. Informed consent should be made in the **absence of pressure or coercion.**[1]

Health officials should also perform ethical analysis from the perspectives of major stakeholders involved in the public health intervention. **Stakeholders** are those for whom a particular environmental health threat will have direct impact.[19] In Vignette 8, although the views of residents of Agresta Ranch should be considered, the issue of risk to the community's health is more important.

The most important ethical issue in Vignette 8 would be **risk analysis**. In this example, the risk of spreading mosquito-borne illnesses far exceeds the benefits of improved water detention basin design, if any. An ethical review of public health research and practice should assess the level of risk associated with the intervention.[19] As the manager in this scenario, you would want to provide Jerry additional education regarding risk analysis to improve his professional competence.

***

Public Health Research Ethics Concepts

Public health practitioners conducting research involving human participants should be cognizant of federal regulations governing research involving human participants as well as the underlying ethical principles. In 1974, the Commission for the Protection of Human Subjects in Biomedical and Behavioral Research published the **Belmont Report**, which set forth three ethical principles that formed the basis of federal regulations pertaining to human participants research: (1) respect for persons, (2) beneficence, and (3) justice.[22] **Respect for persons** is the obligation to treat participants as autonomous agents and obtain informed consent (ensure they agree to the risks, benefits, and alternatives) to participating in research. **Beneficence** refers to protecting the well-being of research participants and ensuring the benefits of research are greater than the risks. The opposite concept is maleficence, which is defined as any action that decreases the welfare of any research participant. **Justice** asks whether the benefits and burdens are distributed fairly (distributive justice) and whether affected groups have the opportunity to participate in making decisions (procedural justice).

If public health practitioners do not adhere to ethics and regulations governing research involving human participants, individuals involved may experience physical risks (e.g., adverse reaction to an antibiotic used in a clinical trial during a meningitis outbreak) or psychosocial risks (e.g., stigma and discrimination).

***

Vignette 9: *Dr. Yang, a scientific expert in human genetics, seeks to examine the genetic underpinnings of disease. He contacts the Pima Nation, a tribe of Native Americans, and tells tribal leaders that he wishes to conduct research examining genetic components of diabetes. Tribal leaders agree. Dr. Yang begins his research by collecting blood samples and medical information from members of the Pima Tribe, telling research participants that they are part of a diabetes research study. Dr. Yang then uses the tribe's blood and medical information for research on schizophrenia.*

What is an example of a negative outcome that may result from Dr. Yang's additional studies?

The Pima Tribe may experience the negative outcome of discrimination as a result of the additional research Dr. Yang conducted without their specific consent. Vignette 9 may be viewed through the lens of the infamous Tuskegee Syphilis Study, the symbol of unethical research conduct with human beings.[19] **Discrimination** refers to an unfair difference in treatment.[23] A related concept is **stigma**, which refers to negative attitudes of associating a trait with a group or individual.[23] Investigators conducting research involving discrete populations, such as Native American tribes and racial, religious, or ethnic minorities, should exercise caution not to overstate implications of their research (e.g., people X are more prone to mental illness) to avoid discrimination or stigmatization of these groups.

***

Ethical Theories to Support Public Health Research, Practice, and Policy

Public health practitioners and policymakers rely upon a number of ethical theories to support public health interventions that include concepts such as utilitarianism, communitarianism, and liberalism.[19]

***

Vignette 10: *Bernice's state representative has asked that she weigh in on whether to amend the state's motorcycle helmet law to allow motorcycle riders aged 21 years and older to ride without a helmet, provided they have $20,000 in medical insurance. She knows that her representative responds well to economic arguments. Using evidence that shows that helmet-less motorcycle riding costs the state millions of dollars more in nonmedical costs, including lost worker productivity, Bernice wants to advocate against the amendment to the mandatory motorcycle helmet law.*

In Vignette 10, utilitarian ethical theory would argue that motorcycle riders should wear helmets because experts have conducted scientific studies that show that wearing helmets saves lives and reduces costs. **Utilitarianism** promotes the goal of the "greatest good for the greatest number" with less concern for individual rights than for social benefit.[19]

On the other hand, **liberalism** focuses on individual rights and freedom to choose. Liberalism ethical theory—unlike the political term used in the United States—seeks to guarantee individual freedom without state infringement on personal choice.[19] In Vignette 10, some groups may disfavor motorcycle helmet laws on the basis that the law interferes with the individual's right to choose whether or not to wear a helmet.

Communitarian theory maintains that individuals are ultimately inseparable from community life and that no one person and no one community can ever be completely self-determining.[19] Communitarianism recognizes that human beings need both autonomy and social relationships. A communitarian approach to this issue focuses not only on the individual's direct benefit from wearing a helmet but also on the benefit that the individual enjoys as a member of a community that reduces motorcycle-related injuries and deaths. While motorcycle riders have a duty to protect themselves in such a way as to not impose a burden on the public, this ethical principal is not as strong as utilitarianism to make the economic argument.

***

Ethical Principles for Building Community Trust

Public health codes of ethics ensure effective trust building with communities that public health organizations, practitioners, and researchers serve.[18] Sustainable public health policy requires **public trust**, and measures that employ force or command without reason may undermine public trust in public health initiatives.[9] Public health professionalism includes a **fiduciary duty** to truth telling and transparency.

***

Vignette 11: *A state health department has just received funding from a for-profit pharmaceutical company to pilot innovative HIV prevention education and needle exchange for drug users in the community. The health department hosted a community forum where some community members complained that providing clean syringes is immoral and a conflict of interest. These community members suggested that the funds should be used for domestic abuse prevention, as women in these circumstances have a higher risk of HIV infection. Other community members argued that there is no evidence that women in abusive relationships have a higher risk of HIV infection. The community is asking that the state health department provide justification for one particular public health action.*

Which approach would help justify the decision of the state health department?

To justify the HIV prevention education and needle exchange for drug users program, the state public health department should provide the community with the information regarding HIV prevention and HIV risk factors. In addition, the state public health department could acknowledge the need to develop a variety of approaches to HIV prevention and domestic violence prevention in order to respect diverse values, beliefs, and cultures in the community. However, because of financial or other resource constraints, the health department may need to choose among several potential strategies, which would involve priority setting. **Priority setting** is a component of health planning that involves the community in decisions related to allocation of scarce resources.[24]

Reaching publicly acceptable decisions also requires considerable deliberation and consensus-building with community members. In Vignette 11, the state health department sought community input regarding the decision by listening and speaking to the community, a public health ethics concept called **reciprocity**.[18] When this communication is truthful, practitioners maintain the ability of public health institutions to effectively serve the communities, a professional ethics concept called **fiduciary duty**.[25]

Finally, public health practitioners should also assess whether any conflict of interest would be implicated by a certain course of action. **Conflicts of interest** occur when the professional actions regarding a primary interest are influenced by a secondary interest.[23] In Vignette 11, the pharmaceutical company does not have a conflict of interest in this example because they are trying to prevent HIV and reduce the need for their drugs. A potential conflict of interest may exist when a public health department employee is an owner or somehow connected with an organization that is regulated by the department. Should conflicts of interest exist, public health organizations, practitioners, and researchers should make them explicit to the public to maintain community trust. Not concealing information is a public health ethic concept called **transparency**.[18]

***

CONCLUSION

This chapter reviewed how public health professionals apply law and ethics in their efforts to keep populations healthy. Legal tension exists between the government's power to protect community health and the limitations on those powers to protect individual rights. In the situations in which the power or duty to act is not clear, the principles of ethical analysis will help you make the most appropriate decision in research, practice, and policy development. Using concepts presented in this chapter, you will be able to advise your colleagues and your community on critical public health law and ethics issues, such as health data regulations, conflicts of interest, social justice, and health disparities.

REFERENCES

1. Gostin LO. *Public Health Law: Power, Duty, Restraint.* 2nd ed. Berkeley, CA: University of California Press; 2008.

2. Centers for Disease Control and Prevention. Public Health Law 101. 2012. Available at: https://www.cdc.gov/phlp/publications/phl_101.html. Accessed April 21, 2018.

3. US Const, art VI.

4. *South Dakota v Dole*, 483 US 203 (1987).

5. National Minimum Drinking Age, 23 USC §158.

6. *National Federation of Independent Businesses v Sebelius*, 567 US 519 (2012).

7. 45 CFR §160 (2002).

8. 45 CFR §164 (2002).

9. Mariner WK, Annas GJ. *Public Health Law.* 2nd ed. New Providence, NJ: Matthew Bender & Company; 2014.

10. 45 CFR §164.512[b] (2003).

11. US Department of Health and Human Services. Health information privacy: when does the privacy rule allow covered entities to disclose protected health information to law

enforcement officials? 2013. Available at: https://www.hhs.gov/hipaa/for-professionals/faq/505/what-does-the-privacy-rule-allow-covered-entities-to-disclose-to-law-enforcement-officials/index.html. Accessed April 21, 2018.

12. *In the Matter of Miguel M.*, 17 NY 3d 37 (2011).

13. *Jacobson v Massachusetts*, 197 US 11 (1905).

14. *Zucht v King*, 260 US 74 (1922).

15. Public Health Service Act, 42 CFR §70.

16. *City of Newark v JS*, 652 A.2d 265 (1993).

17. United Nations. The Universal Declaration of Human Rights. 1948. Available at: http://www.un.org/en/documents/udhr. Accessed April 21, 2018.

18. Public Health Leadership Society. Principles of the Ethical Practice of Public Health, Version 2.2. American Public Health Association. 2002. Available at: https://www.apha.org/-/media/files/pdf/membergroups/ethics/ethics_brochure.ashx?la=en&hash=1E9425A9C96347E42AC0D6B0D2000AA6A8717C3C. Accessed June 14, 2018.

19. Jennings B, Kahn J, Mastroianni A, Parker LS, eds. *Ethics and Public Health: Model Curriculum.* 2003. Available at: https://repository.library.georgetown.edu/bitstream/handle/10822/556779/se0583.pdf?seq. Accessed April 21, 2018.

20. Centers for Disease Control and Prevention. *Community Health and Program Services (CHAPS): Health Disparities Among Racial/Ethnic Populations.* Atlanta, GA: US Department of Health and Human Services; 2008.

21. Bernheim RG, Nieburg P, Bonnie RJ. Ethics and the practice of public health. In: Goodman RA, Hoffman RE, Lopez W, Matthews GW, Rothstein MA, Foster KL, eds. *Law in Public Health Practice.* 2nd ed. New York, NY: Oxford University Press; 2007:110–135.

22. *The Belmont Report.* Washington, DC: The National Commission for the Protection of Human Subjects of Biomedical and Behavioral Research; 1979.

23. Quah SR, Cockerham WC, eds. *International Encyclopedia of Public Health.* 2nd ed. Waltham, MA: Elsevier; 2016.

24. Mays GP. Organization of the public health delivery system. In: Novick LF, Morrow CB, Mays GP, eds. *Public Health Administration: Principles for Population-Based Management.* 2nd ed. Sudbury, MA: Jones & Bartlett Publishers; 2008:69–126.

25. Gostin LO. Introduction: mapping the issues. In: Gostin LO, ed. *Public Health Law and Ethics: A Reader.* 2nd ed. Berkeley, CA: University of California Press; 2010:1–20.

5

Public Health Biology and Human Disease Risk

Jaime A. Corvin, PhD, MSPH, CPH, Thomas Unnasch, PhD, Amy Alman, PhD, Ira Richards, PhD, Karen D. Liller, PhD, Hari H. Venkatachalam, MPH, CPH, and Steven Mlynarek, PhD

INTRODUCTION

As public health advances into the 21st century, an important focus on public health biology is reemerging. This includes our traditional focus on infectious disease, while also advancing public health efforts related to noncommunicable and chronic diseases, nutrition, genetics and genomics, and the cognitive sciences. This chapter will examine the evolution of public health biology and disease risk, outline how biological agents affect health and inform public health laws and regulations, and identify factors that influence infectious and noncommunicable diseases. Specifically, after completion of this chapter, the reader will be able to meet the following tasks:

❏ Assess how biological agents affect human health.
❏ Apply evidence-based biological concepts to inform public health laws, policies, and regulations.
❏ Identify risk factors and modes of transmission for infectious diseases and how these diseases affect both personal and population health.
❏ Identify risk factors for noninfectious diseases and how these issues affect both personal and population health.

MAJOR CONTENT

Biological and Molecular Basis for Public Health

Public health, particularly the field of epidemiology, is based on the premise that health events (or disease) are not random events within the population but that these conditions are more likely to occur as a result of risk factors. Often, these risk factors are not randomly distributed in the population and are, in fact, influenced by biological and social determinants of health.[1] To help us understand disease transmission and how these conditions influence the public's health, epidemiologists have developed **models of disease**

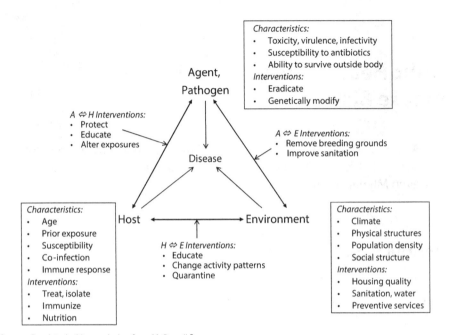

Figure 5-1. The Epidemiologic Triangle Explained

causation. The Epidemiologic Triad, or **Epidemiologic Triangle**, is one of the most commonly used models to illustrate the relationship among an agent, a host, and the environment. Figure 5-1 illustrates the Epidemiologic Triangle. For the condition to occur, the basic elements of causation and an adequate **chain of transmission** (i.e., environmental pathway) must be present.[1]

The Epidemiologic Triangle explains that disease occurs when an outside **agent** (entity that causes disease; can be chemical, physical, or biological) capable of causing the disease interacts with a vulnerable **host** (e.g., susceptible organism, human, animal) in an **environment** (conditions that are not part of the agent and/or host but influence their interaction). The **chain of transmission** of infectious disease helps to illustrate how an infectious agent develops and spreads. The six elements of this chain are elaborated here using the common cold as an example[1,3]:

1. **Causative agent**: Any microorganism that can cause infection (e.g., the common cold virus)
2. **Reservoir or source**: The environment where the agent resides; water sources, feces, bodily secretions (e.g., an individual's nasal cavity)
3. **Portal of exit**: How the agent leaves the reservoir of the host (e.g., when the host sneezes)
4. **Mode of transmission**: How the agent travels to another host; this may be direct or may include an intermediate or indirect contact (e.g., droplets are inhaled by another individual)

5. **Portal of entry**: Where the infectious agent enters a susceptible host (e.g., an opening, including the nose or mouth)
6. **Susceptible host**: Individual or animal that is susceptible to infection (e.g., individual with low immune system)

Public health professionals seek to apply prevention efforts to disrupt any of the pathways of the Epidemiologic Triangle to prevent disease at a population level.

The Risk and Global Burden of Infectious Disease

Infectious diseases represent a declining public health burden throughout most of the developing world. This is primarily attributable to improvements in public health that directly target these diseases. Some of the most effective health interventions that have been developed over the past century, including clean water, sanitation, and vaccination, have been effective in targeting infectious diseases and have resulted in dramatic improvements in the population as a whole. However, making major inroads into reducing the burden of infectious diseases in the developing world has occurred much more slowly.

Historically, the burden of infectious diseases was measured by using gross mortality rates. However, many infectious diseases, while exhibiting low mortality rates, result in severe morbidity. The metric **disability adjusted life years (DALYs)** is used to take the morbidity as well as mortality into account when one is calculating the overall burden of disease. DALY calculations are often used as a way to determine the cost-effectiveness of various disease interventions. Measuring the cost per DALY is one way to help programs most effectively prioritize spending on disease interventions. For example, a recent study has shown that interventions targeting malaria and some of the neglected tropical diseases (particularly onchocerciasis) are among the most cost-effective ways to improve the health of populations in the developing world.[4]

Modes of Infectious Disease Transmission

Pathogens can be transmitted through a variety of mechanisms. From simplest to most complex, these are as follows[5]:

1. **Direct contact**: This is the simplest way a pathogen can be transmitted. Transmission requires direct contact with tissues, blood, bodily fluids, or secretions from an infected individual or animal. Ebola virus is a good example of a pathogen transmitted through direct contact. Sexually transmitted pathogens also fall into this category.
2. **Indirect contact**: Indirect contact is similar to direct contact, but direct contact with bodily fluids or secretions is not required. The pathogen may be capable of surviving for varying periods of time on objects or surfaces and can be transmitted when an infected person comes into contact with the contaminated surface or object. Inanimate

objects capable of transmitting a pathogen are known as **fomites**. Pathogens capable of being transmitted in this way include the influenza virus and norovirus.

3. **Airborne**: Several pathogens are capable of being transmitted through the air. This is usually accomplished through droplets expelled from an infected individual from a cough or sneeze. The effectiveness of pathogen transmission by an airborne route is a function of the droplet size necessary to carry the pathogen and the susceptibility of the pathogen to desiccation. Examples of airborne-transmitted pathogens include those that cause influenza, measles, and severe acute respiratory syndrome (SARS).

4. **Water- and soil-borne**: Pathogens transmitted in this manner can survive for relatively long periods in either soil or water and are transmitted when an individual ingests contaminated soil, food, or water samples. *Vibrio cholerae* and *Necator americanus* (hookworm) are good examples of such pathogens.

5. **Vector-borne**: Vector-borne pathogens represent perhaps the most significant class of infectious agents worldwide. They fall into many classes: viruses, bacteria, unicellular eukaryotes, and multicellular invertebrates (worms). Insects are the most common vectors of infectious disease, but many other classes of organisms can serve as vectors, including ticks, snails, and copepods (water fleas). Table 5-1 summarizes the most common vector-borne diseases and their vectors.

Vectors for pathogens can be either mechanical or biological. Pathogens transmitted by mechanical vectors do not infect the vector. They are just carried from host to host by the vector. House flies are a good example of a mechanical vector, as they can carry a variety of infectious agents including those that cause food poisoning and trachoma. However, biological vectors are far more common and dangerous. In a biological vector, the pathogen is able to infect and develop within the vector, generally amplifying its numbers, resulting in far more efficient transmission than transmission by a mechanical vector. However, biological transmission requires that the pathogen be capable of infecting and developing within both an invertebrate and human host, which are very different environments. Table 5-1 lists agents and vectors for common vector-borne diseases.[5]

The key metric that determines if a given insect can serve as an efficient biological vector is its vectorial capacity.[6] Vectorial capacity is determined by several variables and can be calculated by using the following formula:

$$V = \left(\frac{ma^2 p^n b}{-\ln p} \right)$$

In this formula, V is the overall vectorial capacity; m is the density (number of vectors per acre) of the vector; a is the probability the vector will feed on the vertebrate host of interest for the pathogen (in public health this is generally humans); and p is the daily survival probability (the chance that an individual insect will live to see another day).

Table 5-1. Agents and Vectors for Common Vector-Borne Diseases

Disease	Causative Agent	Vector(s)	Common Name	Transmission
Malaria	Plasmodium falciparum, P. malariae, P. ovale, P. knowlesi, P. vivax	Anopheles spp. (A. gambiae most common)	Mosquito	Biological
Lymphatic filariasis (elephantiasis)	Wuchereria bancrofti, Brugia malayi, B. timori	Culex quinquefasciatus, Anopheles spp., Mansonia spp.	Mosquito	Biological
Breakbone fever	Dengue virus	Aedes aegypti, Aedes albopictus	Mosquito	Biological
Yellow fever	Yellow fever virus	Aedes aegypti, Aedes albopictus	Mosquito	Biological
West Nile fever	West Nile virus	Culex spp. (quinquefasciatus/pipiens and tarsalis most common in United States)	Mosquito	Biological
Zika	Zika virus	Aedes aegypti	Mosquito	Biological
Trachoma	Chlamydia trachomatis	Musca domestica	Housefly	Mechanical
Plague	Yersinia pestis	Xenopsylla cheopis	Flea	Biological
Lyme disease	Borrelia burgdorferi	Ixodes scapularis	Deer tick	Biological
Rocky Mountain spotted fever	Rickettsia rickettsii	Dermacentor variabilis	Tick	Biological
Sleeping sickness	Trypanosoma brucei	Glossina spp.	Tsetse fly	Biological
Leishmaniasis	Leishmania donovani, L. infantum, L. chagasi	Lutzomyia spp.	Sandflies	Biological
River blindness	Onchocerca volvulus	Simulium spp. (major vector S. damnosum in Africa)	Black flies	Biological
Guinea worm	Dracunculus medinensis	Cyclops spp.	Water fleas (copepods)	Biological
Bilharzia	Schistosoma mansoni, S. japonicum, S. haematobium	Biomphalaria spp., Bulinus spp., Oncomelania spp.	Snails	Biological

Source: Based on Moore.[5]

n is the extrinsic incubation period. This is the time in days that it takes from when a vector insect takes an infected blood meal for the pathogen to develop in the insect to the point where it can be transmitted to another susceptible host. Or, simply put, n is the time it takes for an **infected** vector to become **infectious**. Finally, b is the competence of the vector. This can be thought of as the proportion of vectors that take up the pathogen that actually become infectious.[7]

Infectious disease modeling involves models that can be very useful tools for public health professionals attempting to control epidemics. While these models are not necessarily very accurate predictors of the course an epidemic will take,[8] they can be very useful in identifying **drivers** of a model or the variables that have a disproportionate effect on the predicted outcomes. Drivers are important, as they can direct one toward interventions that will be very effective in controlling an outbreak or help identify interventions that will have little effect on an epidemic, and thus should not be pursued.[9]

In infectious diseases, the key parameter that determines if a pathogen will cause an epidemic or will never gain a foothold is the basic reproductive number, or **R**. When a pathogen enters a totally susceptible population, transmission is as efficient as it will ever be. The basic reproductive number in such a situation is designated the $\mathbf{R_0}$, or R at time zero. R is an estimate of the average number of new cases of an infection that the initial infection is capable of spawning. If R is one, every case of an infection will result in on average just one new case, and the infection will be at equilibrium. If the R value is greater than 1, the incidence of the infection will increase, and an epidemic will result. If R is less than one, the infection will disappear from the population. In general, R will decrease as an infection begins to run through a population. This is because people will become immune and start to figure out ways to protect themselves from becoming infected.[10]

Almost all infectious disease models are based on a similar foundation, known as the SEIR model. SEIR stands for **susceptible, exposed, infectious,** and **recovered.** Every day, a certain proportion of the susceptible population will become exposed to the pathogen and move into the exposed group. Similarly, every day, some of the exposed people will develop enough of a titer of the pathogen to become infectious and capable of infecting susceptible people. Finally, every day, some proportion of the people in the infectious group will recover from their infection and move into the recovered group. Although this seems simple, in fact, SEIR models can become complex quite quickly, as they must also account for those who die, recover, become immune, or enter into a carrier state.[9]

Adaptive immunity to infectious conditions can be active or passive and may be either naturally or artificially acquired. As an example of naturally acquired immunity, an infant may receive antibodies that may pass from the mother to the fetus via the placenta or breast milk. This is also immunity that was passively acquired. Conversely, an individual may be exposed to an infectious agent. The body produces antibodies and the individual recovers from the infection resulting in naturally acquired (active) immunity. Artificially acquired immunity includes vaccination. **Vaccination** is the administration of antigenic material (a vaccine) that stimulates an immune response. This is the safest, most effective way to provide immunity to infectious conditions. Vaccinated individuals not only protect themselves but also help to protect the health of all, as they cannot pass the disease to someone who is not immune. However, some individuals, including the very young or the immunocompromised, cannot be vaccinated. These individuals rely on **herd immunity**, or the concept that indirect protections from infectious disease occur when a large portion of a population is immune to infection. Epidemiologists caution that a certain percentage of the population must be immunized to prevent the spread of the disease. Although this threshold varies by disease, depending on risk of infection and mode of disease transmission, between 80% and 85% of the population must be immunized to prevent the spread of disease, and as high as 95% for highly infectious airborne diseases such as measles.[3]

Global Burden of Noncommunicable Diseases

Noncommunicable diseases are mostly chronic and place a tremendous burden on public health and health care systems because of the need for primary prevention programs, a robust health delivery infrastructure, skilled health care workforce, and the long duration of treatment.[4] According to the World Health Organization, chronic diseases accounted for 68% of all deaths worldwide in 2012.[6] The majority of these deaths (82%) are attributable to cardiovascular diseases, cancers, chronic respiratory diseases, and diabetes.[6] The burden of noncommunicable disease is expected to significantly increase over the next two decades, particularly for low- and low-middle–income countries.[8] The changing demography of global populations has led to chronic diseases surpassing infectious diseases as the leading causes of morbidity and mortality.[11]

Population aging has resulted in a shift in the age distribution in both wealthy and poor countries with larger proportions of older individuals who are at increased risk for chronic disease.[8] Chronic diseases that are strongly age-dependent, such as stroke, chronic obstructive pulmonary disease, diabetes, and dementia, will increase as the relative population of older individuals increases.[12] Decreases in fertility coupled with increased life expectancy have contributed to a shift in the median age in many countries that is expected to increase over time.[8,12] Gender differences in life expectancy, prevalence of disease, risk factors, and susceptibility play an important role in future disease burden.[12]

Successes in health care and other programs targeting acute causes of morbidity and mortality, such as infectious and nutritional diseases, have greatly increased the number of individuals living into adulthood.[8,12] Antibiotic use and vaccination programs have been extremely successful at reducing mortality from infectious diseases, but coupled with the increased prevalence of modifiable risk factors for noncommunicable diseases, such as unhealthy diet, tobacco and alcohol use, and physical inactivity, chronic diseases have become the leading cause of mortality globally.[8] In higher-income countries, as treatment improves for chronic diseases and mortality declines, as has been seen for cardiovascular disease, the prevalence of the disease increases as more individuals survive longer resulting in a significant impact on the population burden of the disease.[12] In low- and middle-income countries, mortality from chronic diseases occurs at younger ages than in high-income countries.[8,12,13]

In addition, the role of **human genetics and genomics** cannot be overlooked. Human genetics focuses on how genes influence disease and behaviors. Today, public health works to apply advances in genetics to understand disease conditions and prevent disease. There are numerous examples of how public health genetics inform health outcomes. Traditional examples include reproductive technologies such as prenatal or carrier screening and newborn screening. However, this field is evolving rapidly and more recent efforts have focused on genetic susceptibility screening and pharmacogenetics.

Many human diseases are associated with genetic defects. Defects can occur as **single gene defects**, which are known as point mutations, and **cytogenetic defects**, which are a result of chromosomal abnormalities. Physical defects may arise during embryonic development. These diseases are called **teratogenic** and the external factors that cause them are called teratogens. **Teratogens** fall under the following categories[5]:

1. **Ionizing radiation:** Gamma or x-rays; this may cause problems with eyes, microcephaly, or intellectual disabilities
2. **Chemicals**
   a. Accutane: Commonly used in the treatment of acne; when used during pregnancy can result in birth defects
   b. Alcohol: May cause fetal alcohol syndrome when consumed during pregnancy
   c. Cigarette smoke: Associated with low birth weight, stillbirth, or miscarriage
   d. Dioxin: Group of chemically related compounds called persistent organic pollutants, which break down slowly, are highly toxic, and are linked to cancer, reproductive issues, and development problems
   e. Thalidomide: A sedative used widely in the 1960s that resulted in phocomelia (the absence of long bones in the legs and arms)
3. **Pathogens**
   a. Rubella: Virus that crosses the placental barrier, causing congenital defects
   b. Syphilis: A sexually transmitted disease that produces microcephaly and intellectual disabilities
   c. Toxoplasmosis: A disease that results from infection with the *Toxoplasma gondii* parasite; infection linked to undercooked contaminated meat, exposure to infected cat feces, and mother-to-child transmission

Most teratogens affect the embryo during **organogenesis**, a critical stage of early development when tissues and organs are formed.

The shift toward an increasing global burden of noncommunicable disease is called the **epidemiologic transition**.[8,12,14–18] Omran proposed that this transition consisted of three stages of transition[16]:

1. The age of pestilence and famine
2. The age of receding pandemics
3. The age of degenerative and man-made diseases

Others have added additional stages:

4. The delay of disease until advanced age[18]
5. The social upheaval and war—resurgence of diseases from earlier stages[18]

There are challenges to addressing this increase in noncommunicable disease, including our relative lack of understanding of the etiology of these diseases. Researchers use conceptual frameworks to address these challenges and to improve knowledge of risk factors and to design interventions.[17] Because of the chronic nature of these diseases and their appearance later in life, increasing evidence suggests that exposures throughout life play an important role in the disease process.

Many factors contribute to noncommunicable diseases. **Ecobiologic** factors include those that are specific to the host as well as to the environment, such as air pollution. **Socioeconomic** factors are social and economic factors that influence disease. Some medical and public health systems also contribute to disease. In many poor countries, the health care system is focused on care for acute conditions and there is a lack of resources to tackle preventive and chronic care necessary to effectively combat noncommunicable diseases.[8,19,20] Even in middle-income or more wealthy countries, lack of health insurance and costs of health care, limited access to preventive care, and changing behavior have proved daunting.

While global rates of noncommunicable diseases are increasing, not all countries, or even regions within countries, are in the same period of the epidemiologic transition at the same time.[18] The World Health Organization's Global Action Plan for the Prevention and Control of Noncommunicable Diseases 2013–2020 calls for a 25% relative reduction in premature mortality attributable to the four main noncommunicable diseases (cardiovascular diseases, cancers, chronic respiratory diseases, and diabetes) by 2025 (relative to mortality in 2010).[21] Efforts to monitor progress toward the goal by reviewing vital registration system data and country or regional characteristics have worked to identify regions with continued high prevalence of the disease. Age-standardized mortality rates can be compared between regions, and analyses can be performed to identify characteristics of regions with high prevalence.[22]

Regions where rheumatic heart disease remains highly prevalent are those with poor or no access to health care, particularly access to penicillin to effectively treat the infection and to provide secondary prevention to prevent sequelae. Also, low education and income contribute to this disease.[22,23] Echocardiography-based screening can identify silent cases of the disease to better characterize the prevalence and to identify cases needing medical or surgical treatment. However, availability of this screening is dependent upon sufficient resources.[22,23]

Availability of **antibiotic prophylaxis** to prevent acute rheumatic fever after a sore throat and to prevent disease recurrence, coupled with **socioeconomic development that improves hygiene, access to medical care, and living conditions**, would lead to dramatic reductions of rheumatic heart disease in regions where the disease is still highly prevalent.[23]

Injuries and Violence

Although not considered a noninfectious disease, injuries and violence are considered serious public health problems that need to be addressed. Injuries are the leading cause of death for Americans between the ages of 1 and 45 years and a source of a great number of deaths internationally. They are the leading cause of death for children and adults in the United States. According to the National Center for Injury Prevention and Control (NCIPC) at the Centers for Disease Control and Prevention (CDC), injuries (unintentional) and violence (homicide, suicide, other violent acts) can affect us all, regardless of age, race, or economic status; however, certain injuries and violence do show increased prevalence in particular populations and in those with lower socioeconomic status. It is true that deaths are only the tip of the iceberg as millions of people are injured and survive. Many are faced with life-long mental, physical, and financial problems. Also, according to the NCIPC, more than 200,000 Americans die from violence and injuries each year—nearly one person every three minutes. In addition, more than 3 million people are hospitalized, and more than 27 million people are treated in emergency departments as a result of violence and injuries each year. Violence and injuries cost the United States more than $600 billion each year in medical care and lost productivity.[24]

Whereas motor vehicle injuries used to be the leading cause of death for children and young adults, this changed for adults in the early 2000s as the number of poisoning and overdose deaths became greater, largely attributable to the rapid increase in opioid use.[25] Drug overdose deaths and opioid-involved deaths continue to increase in the United States with the greatest number of drug overdose deaths (66%) involving an opioid.[25] According to the NCIPC, in 2016, the number of overdose deaths involving opioids (including prescription opioids and heroin) was five times higher than in 1999. From 2000 to 2016, more than 600,000 people died from drug overdoses in the United States. On average, 115 Americans die every day from an opioid overdose. Strategies to combat this epidemic are ongoing but focus on stricter prescribing requirements for physicians, patient and physician education, use of prescription drug monitoring programs, medication-assisted therapy, use of naloxone for overdose reversal, and more.[25]

Over the years, successful injury prevention efforts have addressed strategies that include education, engineering change, and enforcement of laws and policies. The Haddon Matrix, which utilizes host, agent, and environmental factors (physical and sociocultural) assessed over time (pre-event, event, and post-event), has been used to develop strategies along with several behavioral science theories and models that have been used to plan and evaluate injury prevention programs.[26]

Evidence-Based Biological Concepts to Inform Public Health Laws, Policies, and Regulations

The physical and social environments are critical to individual and community health. The physical environment comprises **air**, **water**, and **soil** through which exposure to **biologic** (e.g., disease organisms present in food and water, insect and animal allergens), **chemical** (e.g., air pollutants, toxic wastes, pesticides, volatile organic compounds [VOCs]), or **physical** (e.g., noise, ionizing and nonionizing radiation) agents may occur, while the social environment includes the **built space** (e.g., housing, transportation, land use and development) and the industry or agriculture in which exposures to harmful agents, work stress, injury, or violence may occur. As the population continues to expand, protecting the environment requires an understanding of the factors that ensure our air is safe to breathe, the water is safe to drink, the land is free from toxicants, and waste is managed well. This requires effective oversight through the development and enforcement of laws, policies, and regulations.[27]

Air Quality

Our air is composed of 78.1% nitrogen, 20.9% oxygen, and 0.9% argon. The remaining 0.1% is made up of carbon dioxide, neon, helium, and methane. The **US Environmental Protection Agency's (EPA's) National Ambient Air Quality Standards (NAAQS)** set the limits for six primary criteria air pollutants that are revised every five years. It is the responsibility of the states to ensure new NAAQS are met.[27] The six primary air pollutants are the following:

1. **Sulfur dioxide (acid rain)**: Sulfur dioxide causes respiratory effects particularly in people with asthma and other susceptible populations.
2. **Nitrogen oxides (smog, acid rain)**: Nitrogen oxides have been linked to respiratory effects. They particularly can affect people with asthma.
3. **Carbon monoxide**: Carbon monoxide reduces the blood's ability to carry oxygen to body tissues. It can affect those with cardiovascular conditions.
4. **Ozone**: Ozone causes airway irritation, coughing, and difficulty breathing. It can affect those with chronic obstructive pulmonary disease (COPD) or asthma.

5. **Lead**: Lead is a metal that occurs naturally. It can cause neurological effects in children and can also affect kidney, immune, development, and reproductive systems.
6. **Particulate matter**: Particulates measure smaller than 10 micrometers. This category includes both PM_{10} and $PM_{2.5}$. Both can cause respiratory effects.

There has been much discussion about the role of ozone and health. Ozone exists either at the ground (surface) level or in the stratosphere. There is no, or very little, transmission of ozone from one level to another. Ozone that exists in the Earth's stratosphere absorbs most of the sun's ultraviolet (UVB) radiation. This region contains high concentrations of ozone (O_3) compared with other parts of the atmosphere, yet this concentration is still small in relation to other gases found in the stratosphere. **Atmospheric ozone**, therefore, has a positive effect on human health. **Ground-level ozone,** however, is a principal component of smog. As a result of the chemical reactions between VOCs and nitrogen, ground-level ozone has been found to be harmful to human health and responsible for aging lung tissue, reducing resistance to colds, and breathing problems.[27]

Specifically, biological effects of ground-level ozone exposure include respiratory and central nervous system effects and have been linked to increased respiratory morbidity outcomes, central nervous system impairment resulting in morbidity, disruption of neurotransmitters, decreased motor activity, impairments to short- and long-term memory, disruption of sleep patterns, and histological signs of neurodegeneration. On the basis of the well-established evidence of changes in the biology of the respiratory system and extensive evidence of the effects of ozone on public health and welfare, on October 1, 2015, the EPA strengthened the guidelines and reduced the NAAQS acceptable level of ground-level ozone to 70 parts per billion (ppb) or 0.07 parts per million (ppm).[5,27]

For workers, The Occupational Safety and Health Administration (OSHA) Web site cites several American Conference of Governmental Industrial Hygienists (ACGIH) guidelines for ozone in the workplace with exposure not to exceed[5,27]:

- 0.2 ppm for no more than 2 hours exposure
- 0.1 ppm for 8 hours per day exposure doing light work
- 0.08 ppm for 8 hours per day exposure doing moderate work
- 0.05 ppm for 8 hours per day exposure doing heavy work

Climate Change

The Earth's average temperature has increased by 1.5°F in the past 100 years, an increase that is expected to continue. Current indicators of climate change include changes in weather patterns and rising global temperatures, increases in surface temperatures of the oceans, and melting of glaciers and polar icecaps. These have resulted in changes in disease patterns and risk, including increases in tick populations and Lyme disease and increases in asthma rates. The source of this increase in temperature is emissions of greenhouse gases.[27]

Greenhouse gases have been created by humans and are the largest driver of climate change. The primary greenhouse gases found in Earth's atmosphere include carbon dioxide, methane, nitrous oxide, ozone, and water vapor.[5]

Water Quality

The earth's water is made up of 97.5% salt water and 2.5% fresh water (68.7% of which is frozen, 30.1% is groundwater, and 1.2% is surface water). Water quality is influenced by droughts, which can lower the water table, or flooding, which can result in water pollution. Sources of water pollution are either[5,27]

- **Point source**: Pollution that comes from a discrete source such as a factory, hazardous waste site, or landfill. The National Pollutant Discharge Elimination System Permit aims to regulate the amount and type of discharge eliminated in public water systems in an effort to prevent pollution of our waters.
- **Nonpoint source**: Pollution from a diffuse source. This includes runoff, which may come from agriculture sources, construction, urban streets, or mines and may also result from airborne pollutant fallout.

Drinking water standards are regulated by the EPA and include legally enforceable standards that apply only to public water systems. Several pathogens are regulated by the EPA, including the following[27]:

- *Cryptosporidium*, a single-cell protozoan found in surface waters contaminated by sewage and animal waste, which is resistant to chlorine treatment;
- *Giardia lamblia*, a single-cell protozoan found in soil, food, or water contaminated with feces of infected humans or animals;
- *Legionella*, a bacteria discovered after a 1976 outbreak at an American Legion convention in Philadelphia, Pennsylvania, that is naturally in the environment but becomes a health risk if it becomes aerosolized and inhaled, resulting in a lung infection; and
- **Enteric viruses,** including norovirus and rotavirus.

Steps for Water Treatment

Drinking water is vulnerable to contamination and so requires treatment to ensure quality and safety. Public drinking water systems use various methods of treatment to ensure the safety of our water supply. The most common steps are outlined in Figure 5-2 and include[28]

1. **Coagulation and flocculation**: During these first steps in water treatment, chemicals with a positive charge are added to the water to neutralize the effects of dirt and other dissolved particles. These dissolved particles and dirt combine with the chemicals to form larger particles called floc.
2. **Sedimentation**: During this phase, floc settles to the bottom of the water.

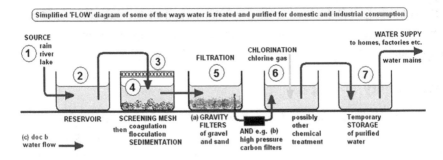

Source: Reprinted with permission from Doc Brown's Chemistry KS4 science GCSE/IGCSE/O Level Chemistry Revision Notes.[29]

Figure 5-2. Water Treatment Diagram

3. **Filtration**: Once the floc settles at the bottom, the clear water on top passes through various filters (sand, gravel, and charcoal), to remove dissolved particles.
4. **Disinfection**: Once filtered, a disinfectant such as chlorine is added to the water to kill any remaining parasites, bacteria, or viruses.[28]

The water treatment diagram in Figure 5-2 illustrates each step.[29]

Sewage Treatment and Disposal

Treatment and proper disposal of sewage is an important aspect of water treatment and has a great deal of public health significance in terms of disease control. This issue is still faced in both developing and developed nations where cross-contamination of drinking water can lead to outbreaks of diarrheal diseases that cause a great deal of morbidity and mortality.[5]

In rural areas in the United States, sewage is still often collected in **septic tanks**, where solids settle, and then the fluid is released into perforated pipes in a drainage field where they are filtered by percolation through the soil. However, such methods are inappropriate in urbanized municipalities. Hence, proper treatment of sewage has become a necessity. The process for treating sewage usually occurs over two steps[5]:

1. **Primary treatment**: A mechanical process that removes 50% to 60% of suspended solids and usually consists of the following:
   a. **Screening**: Removes large solids.
   b. **Grinding**: Reduces solids to uniform size.
   c. **Sedimentation**: Solids are separated in a grit chamber.
   d. **Primary clarification:** Floating scum and settled sludge are dried and disposed.
2. **Secondary treatment:** A biological process that removes 90% to 95% of the suspended solids and usually consists of the following:
   a. **Activated sludge process:** The remaining sewage is oxidized to rapidly break down organic material.
   b. **Secondary clarification**: Afloat scum and settled sludge are dried and disposed.

Sewage treatment can vary among different municipal systems. Some treatment systems only perform primary treatment, while others add an additional step, or **tertiary treatment**, which can consist of disinfection for the purpose of reusing the water for lakes and ponds. **Chlorination** is also often performed on treated sewage as an additional way of controlling disease transmission.

Effectiveness of sewage treatment is often measured by diminishing the **biological oxygen demand** (**BOD**) of the wastewater. **Dissolved oxygen** is often plentiful in natural waterways and helps support the aquatic wildlife. Contamination with organic material, such as that found in sewage, results in breakdown processes that deplete the dissolved oxygen due to the increased BOD of the decomposing organic matter. A sign of such contamination is the presence of dead fish and other aquatic wildlife in natural bodies of water. The BOD of water can easily be checked with a simple chemical test. Each stage of the sewage treatment process reduces the BOD of the wastewater, with primary, secondary, and tertiary treatment reducing BOD by 20% to 30%, 85%, and 99% respectively. Finally, the treated wastewater becomes progressively more aerated as it travels from the point of discharge.[5,30]

Food Safety

To ensure food safety, critical control points are necessary. Time and temperature are the greatest challenges with food safety. Temperatures between **39°F** **and 140°**F are considered to be in the **danger zone.** Handwashing and worker hygiene are also critical. Other factors include cross-contamination, ensuring safe and reputable food sources, and adequate labeling to identify food allergens. When safety protocols are not followed, risk of foodborne illness arises. Foodborne illness results from consuming food or beverages containing harmful microorganisms or chemical contaminants. Although symptoms and incubation vary by pathogen, symptoms tend to include stomach cramping or pain, vomiting, diarrhea, fever, headaches, chills, and body aches. Outbreaks tend to be detected at the local or state level. Health agencies are required to report all cases of foodborne illness to CDC. The Food and Drug Administration (FDA) becomes involved with any outbreak that involves an FDA-regulated product.[5]

Hazard Analysis and Critical Control Points (HACCP) is a preventive measure developed as a systematic approach to the identification, evaluation, and control of food safety hazards. The seven HACCP Principles are as follows[27]:

1. Conduct hazard analysis;
2. Determine critical control points (point at which a measure of control can be applied preventing, eliminating, or reducing hazard to acceptable level);
3. Establish critical limits (the value to which a parameter must be controlled, including time, temperature, physical dimensions, humidity, moisture, pH, etc.);
4. Establish monitoring procedures to allow the opportunity to take corrective action;

5. Establish the corrective action to be taken when monitoring indicates that a critical limit has been exceeded;
6. Establish procedures to verify that the HACCP system is working; and
7. Establish effective record keeping that will document the HACCP system.

Solid Waste

Waste management is a concept developed in the 20th century. Before that time, waste was often discarded in lakes, rivers, oceans, or lands with little regard to the effects on the environment. However, in the early 20th century, processes for waste handling and disposal became widespread in the United States and other developed countries. Today, municipalities are responsible for solid waste disposal, which includes recycling, landfilling, composting, and combustion.[27]

Materials that are unable to be recycled or composted should be deposited in a local landfill to help reduce environmental effects. Landfills comprise the following[27]:

- A bottom liner;
- A system for collecting **leachate**, the water that has passed through the waste and collected contaminates of that waste;
- A cover; and
- An appropriate location to minimize groundwater contamination. Dangers of landfills that are not well constructed include air pollution and groundwater contamination. Federal laws require that the groundwater around landfills be routinely tested and corrective action be taken as necessary.

Hazardous waste is waste that is potentially hazardous to human or environmental health when improperly disposed. Hazardous waste tends to come primarily from (1) hazardous materials in the home including pesticides, cleaning products, painting supplies, and automotive products; (2) medical waste, which may include chemicals, infectious agents, or even radioactive materials; (3) industrial hazardous waste including chemicals, solvents, and heavy metals; (4) radioactive waste; and (5) mining waste including toxic chemicals that result from mining processes.[27]

The Love Canal, located near Niagara Falls, was a toxic waste site that is significant to the field of public health as the incident that helped to illustrate the link between hazardous chemical exposure and the possible influence on human health. When disposal of toxic chemicals, such as halogenated organic compounds, chlorobenzenes, and dioxin, ended in 1952 with the closure of the site, the presence of toxic chemicals was observed near the former site and residents in the area reported high rates of miscarriage, birth defects, and cancer. As a result of the Love Canal incident, the Superfund was created and administered by the EPA. **Superfund regulations** require that responsible parties must assume liability for the cleanup of environmental hazards that they cause.[27]

Deaths attributable to toxic substances in the environment are nothing new. Hippocrates described the symptoms of lead poisoning in 370 BC. **Toxicology** is an underlying principle of environmental health.

Chemical Agents

Chemical agents may be solid, liquid, or gaseous substances that produce harmful effects on a living organism. Table 5-2 lists common toxins, their primary source, common effects, and potential prevention strategies.[5,27]

Routes of exposure: There are three major routes of exposure by which chemicals enter the body[5,27]:

- **Dermal entry** or penetration through the skin,
- **Inhalation** or absorption through the lungs, and
- **Orally** or passage across the walls of the gastrointestinal tract.

The most common route of exposure to chemical agent that leads to toxicity is **inhalation**. Although the human skin, the largest organ of the human body, regularly comes in contact with many chemical agents, it is an extremely effective barrier to chemicals. The lungs provide a much less effective barrier to chemicals.[5,27]

Toxicology is the study of how chemicals cause injury to living cells and whole organisms. **Dose** refers to the amount of the chemical in the body. **Risk** is the probability that harm will be produced under a specific set of conditions. Risk includes the combination of two considerations: the probability or likelihood that an adverse event will occur and the consequences or level of harm that will result if it does[5,27]:

$$\text{Risk} = \text{Toxicity} \times \text{Exposure}$$

The dose–response curve illustrates the change in effect on an organism that is caused by differing levels of exposure (see Figure 5-3). It is assumed that the higher the dose, the greater the effects observed. Deleterious effects are expected to occur after reaching a threshold dose amount. An exception is the **carcinogen rule**. For carcinogens, there is no safe threshold level.[5,27]

Lethal dose is an important measurement in toxicology. Lethal dose 50 (LD_{50}) is the most common measure of acute toxicity. This is a statistical figure denoting the dose level at which 50% of the test population is expected to die.[31]

Acute toxicity is the ability of a substance to do systemic damage as a result of a one-time exposure of a short duration, and **chronic toxicity** includes systemic effects that are produced by long-term and often low-level exposure.[5,27]

Risk assessment is a methodology that assists in evaluating the human health effects and environmental consequences of exposure to chemicals. Just as the dose–response assessment for several chemicals makes it possible to rank them by their relative toxicities,

Table 5-2. Common Environmental Toxins

Toxin	Source	Effect	Prevention Strategy
Phthalates	Plasticizers found in medical and household plastic and metal products (e.g., plastic wrap, liners of food and beverage cans).	Associated with testicular toxicity.	Limiting use of plastic and metal products, reduction of processed food items which contain the toxin.
Dioxin	Byproduct of chlorinated hydrocarbons, paper bleaching, and plastic incineration. Formed by incomplete combustion of wood production and industrial/municipal wastes.	Carcinogenic. Accumulates in tissues and breaks down slowly in the environment. Adverse reproductive and developmental effects, neurological damage, endocrine disruption.	Reducing occupational contact with these substances through careful industrial hygiene protocols.
Polychlorinated biphenyls (PCBs)	Used in electrical transformers and capacitors, hydraulic fluids, plasticizers, and adhesives. Used to coat electrical wires; provide protective coating to lumber, concrete, and metal surfaces.	Bind to thyroid hormones and interfere with normal growth and metabolism. Results in psychomotor development delays in children.	Banned in the United States in the 1970s. Strategies should target old homes and replace old appliances.
Lead	Used in paints, inks, and glazes. Found in gasoline. Can be found in leaching from old pipes.	Slows the maturation of red blood cells in the bone marrow. Inhibits synthesis of hemoglobin. Impairs fertility. Severe cognitive issues over time.	Banned for commercial use in 1978. Strategies should target old homes, remove lead paint.
Organic solvents	Typically exposure comes from occupational contact for those in the medical or electronic industries. Typical exposure is through inhalation.	Can result in spontaneous abortions, birth defects such as cleft palate and lip, CNS and cardiovascular defects in newborns.	Prevention of exposure; improved occupational health in industries where individuals come into contact with organic solvents.
Asbestos	Used in wall insulation and ceilings, around pipes and vents, for heat resistance in shingles.	Human carcinogen, specifically those involving the lining of the lung or abdomen.	Target schools positive for asbestos.
Mercury	Thermometers, batteries, the production of chlorine, and fluorescent light bulbs.	Caused pink disease (1940–50). Slurred speech, difficulty swallowing, ultimately death.	Proper disposal of products that contain mercury.

(Continued)

Table 5-2. (Continued)

Toxin	Source	Effect	Prevention Strategy
Arsenic	Found in pesticides, herbicides, fertilizers, the treatment process of human waste, industrial sources, and volcanic eruptions.	Results in diaphoresis, abdominal pain, muscle spasms, nausea, vomiting, dehydration, anuria, diarrhea, anemia, hypotension, cardiovascular collapse, death.	Prevent usage of pesticides and herbicides near aquifers and sources of drinking water. Test water sources for arsenic.
Biological agents (bacterial, fungal, viral)	Variety of sources: vectors, vehicles, fomite contact, person-to-person, animal-to-person.	Variety of diseases: cholera, influenza, etc.	Decontamination of food products, water, and education on hygiene.
Carbon monoxide	Produced from the incomplete combustion of fossil fuels.	Dizziness, headaches, visual impairment, poor learning ability, limited dexterity, paralysis, death.	Limiting motor vehicle emissions; restricting running vehicles in unventilated spaces.
Nitrogen and sulfur oxides	Combustion of fossil fuels and industrial activity in boilers and automotive engines.	Respiratory illnesses and decreased protection from agent-caused respiratory illnesses.	Maintenance and restrictions on industrial activity.
Secondhand tobacco smoke	Nonsmoker contact with smokers; passive inhalation when the smoker is smoking.	Lung cancer.	Restricting smoking in public spaces.
Ozone	Reaction between sunlight, nitrogen dioxide, and volatile hydrocarbons.	Respiratory infections increase and inflammation of lung tissue.	Enforce EPA standards of ozone .08 ppm. Restrictions for outdoor workers when ozone levels elevated.
Formaldehyde	Found in pressed wood products such as cabinets and furniture.	Irritation of mucous membranes, severe allergic reactions, wheezing, fatigue, and coughing.	Proper ventilation in structures that contain volatile formaldehyde; guidelines to produce minimal formaldehyde-emitting products.
Radon	Natural decay of radium-226, a product of uranium decay. Found in uranium and phosphate ores. Found also in limestone, shale, and granite.	Risk of lung cancer.	Monitoring buildings and homes for radon. Focus on areas with higher concentrations.

Source: Based on Moore.[5]

Note: CNS = central nervous system; EPA = Environmental Protection Agency; ppm = parts per million.

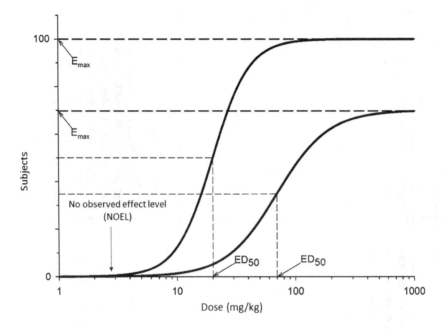

Figure 5-3. The Dose–Response Curve

risk assessments should be used as a tool for the allocation of public health resources aimed toward recognizing, prioritizing, and reducing human health risk and environmental problems.[5,27]

In theory, risk assessments should be recognized for their value and limitations in public health programs and in the making of rational management decisions, which are always based in part on financial considerations. It is the responsibility of public health professionals when communicating risk to present results clearly and accurately so that everyone can hopefully understand the difference between a hazard as described through the risk assessment process and a risk that is only "perceived" as real. There have been serious concerns about the benefits to the public from the extremely costly cleanups of some areas deemed hazardous.[5,27]

In assessing a risk to public health, a progression of steps is necessary[5,27]:

1. **Hazard identification**: Determines if a chemical under exposure conditions likely to occur in humans can cause an increase in the incidence or severity of an adverse health effect. Epidemiologic studies and laboratory animal studies, in vitro tests, and structural and mechanistic comparability with other known chemical hazards are considered.

2. **Dose–response assessment**: The process of characterizing the relationship between the dose of a chemical and the severity and incidence of adverse health effects in an exposed population. It must consider factors such as the duration, frequency, and magnitude of exposure, as well as confounding issues such as age, sex, and lifestyle

factors. This often requires extrapolation from animals to humans and from high to low doses. It is important to note that all substances can, at some level, be harmful to health. As an example, sodium fluoride is good for teeth but, at high levels, causes tooth enamel discoloration; vitamin D is necessary for human health but is toxic when it is more than 10 milligrams per kilogram. Even water at incredibly high doses (which is improbable) can cause hyperhydration and be fatal.[32]

3. **Exposure assessment**: The process of identifying potential exposure routes, specifying an exposed population, and measuring or estimating the magnitude, duration, and frequency of an exposure. Exposures can be estimated with a variety of exposure models and/or assessed by direct measurement.

4. **Risk characterization**: The development of a qualitative, semi-quantitative, or quantitative estimate of the risk associated with a given chemical under a defined exposure scenario(s). The characterization must attempt to encompass multiple populations with varying sensitivities and exposures. Limitations and uncertainties must be identified so that all concerned parties understand the strengths and weaknesses of the risk estimates.

A major challenge to regulatory agencies is the fact that human data are often limited, meaning that inferences concerning risk must be made from animal toxicity studies that use high exposure levels. The question then becomes not what are the exposure levels that pose a toxicity risk but, rather, what are the exposure levels that are more likely to be encountered in the environment on the best day. In addition, humans are exposed to a multitude of chemicals at any given time that may interact with one another in complex and/or unpredictable ways in the body and in the environment.

Federal Laws

Human illness and death related to environmental exposures remain some of the most significant challenges for public health practitioners.[27] Environmental policies have been increasingly designed to protect human health. Current environmental regulation regards protection from environmental hazards as a fundamental human right and increasingly seeks to reduce disparities in health status associated with such exposures.[27]

Myriad agencies—from international, national, state/territorial, and local levels—are responsible for the development and enforcement of environmental health regulations, including the following:

- **World Health Organization (WHO)**: According to its Web site, the overall goal of WHO is to build a better, healthier future for people all over the world. Working through offices in more than 150 countries, WHO staff work side by side with governments and other partners to ensure the highest attainable level of health for all people (see http://www.who.int/about/en).[33]

Table 5-3. Important US Laws Concerning Pollution

Policy	Purpose
Clean Air Act	Provided for the establishment of NAAQS by regulating six classes of air pollutants (lead was added later) or criteria air pollutants, regulated vehicle emissions, and established protocols for regulating other air pollutants (hazardous air pollutants).
Toxic Substances Control Act (TSCA)	Mandated that manufacturers of chemicals develop safety and health data on chemicals and mixtures and required the EPA to regulate substances and mixtures that may pose risk of injury to health or the environment.
Clean Water Act	Renamed in 1977 from the Federal Water Pollution Control Act. Established national standards for waterways and set limits on pollutant discharges.
Comprehensive Environmental Response, Compensation, and Liability Act (CERCLA)	Created with the intent of providing cleanup of existing inactive and abandoned hazardous waste sites through the creation of superfunds. Was strengthened by the Superfund Amendments and Reauthorization Act of 1986.
Noise Control Act of 1972	Act to abate noise in the ambient environment and communities through investigating of sources, controlling noise pollution, and enacting policies.
Nuclear Waste Policy Act	Created in 1982 and delegated responsibility for high-level radioactive waste management to the federal government and designated the US Department of Energy as the agency to coordinate efforts to site, construct, and operate permanent repositories for nuclear waste products.
Federal Water Pollution Control Act of 1972	Original legislation that later was renamed the Clean Water Act of 1972. Established national standards for the nation's waterways and set limits on allowed pollutant discharges.
Safe Drinking Water Acts	Regulated the public drinking water systems. Allowed the EPA to set maximum contaminant levels for water pollutants in drinking water.
Comprehensive Air Quality Act of 1967	First attempt to develop a regional approach for the control of air pollution through the designation of Air Quality Control Regions. Retained oversight of air quality at the level of the states. The Clean Air Act of 1970 ultimately would move power from the level of the states to the level of the federal government, specifically the EPA.
Resource Conservation and Recovery Act	Similar to CERCLA but prevents hazardous waste problems at active sites. Identifies hazardous waste under the criteria of ignitability, corrosivity, reactivity, and toxicity, and tracks from generation, transportation, treatment, storage, and disposal in a cradle-to-grave system. It also mandated accurate record keeping of all these steps of hazardous waste management.
Emergency Planning and Community Right-to-Know Act	Required private and public facilities to report publicly their waste production for hazardous wastes.
Hazardous Materials Transportation Act	Provided guidance on the transportation of hazardous materials and placed authority within the Department of Transportation. States most abide by these federal regulations but can place more stringent provisions. It covers any materials that are capable of creating an unreasonable risk to health.

(Continued)

Table 5-3. (Continued)

Policy	Purpose
Pollution Prevention Act	Focused on the remediation and treatment of pollution, rather than prevention. Any pollution that cannot be prevented should be recycled, treated, and disposed of in a way that does not harm the environment. Placed role of prevention with the states and provides financial support for such activities.

Source: Based on Moore.[5]

Note: EPA = Environmental Protection Agency; NAAQS = National Ambient Air Quality Standards.

- **European Environment Agency (EEA):** According to its Web site, the EEA provides sound, independent information on the environment for those involved in developing, adopting, implementing. and evaluating environmental policy, and also for the general public (see https://www.eea.europa.eu).[34]
- **US Environmental Protection Agency (EPA):** The mission of the EPA is to protect human health and the environment. The EPA was established in response to public demand for cleaner water, air, and land.[35]
- **National Institute for Occupational Safety and Health (NIOSH)** and **Occupational Safety and Health Administration (OSHA):** NIOSH is the federal agency responsible for conducting research and making recommendations related to the prevention of workplace injury and illness. OSHA sets and enforces standards for workplace chemical exposures in the United States.[36,37]
- **Agency for Toxic Substances and Disease Registry (ATSDR):** ATSDR is an agency of the US Department of Health and Human Services that serves the public by using the best science to inform the public and prevent harmful exposures related to toxic substances. ATSDR is the principal federal public health agency involved in hazardous waste issues.[38]
- **National Institute of Environmental Health Sciences (NIEHS):** The mission of NIEHS is to reduce the burden of human illness related to environmental causes through the understanding of environmental factors, individual susceptibility, and age.[39]

Federal laws help regulate what our safest maximum exposures should be to potentially hazardous agents. Environmental policies and laws follow the same processes outlined in Chapter 4, "Law and Ethics." Although the number of federal laws are numerous and diverse, Table 5-3 outlines environmental law and policies that are of critical importance to public health.

PRACTICE QUESTIONS

1. The Zika virus is transmitted primarily by *Aedes aegypti*, the yellow fever mosquito. *Ae. aegypti* is a tropical mosquito whose range in the United States is limited to the southern states. However, the Asian tiger mosquito, *Aedes albopictus* is a potential vector for

Zika, and it has a much broader range in the United States than does *Ae. aegypti*. Which of the following would NOT be an effective method to determine if *Ae. albopictus* might become an important vector for Zika virus in the United States?

    a. Test those infected with Zika to determine which species of mosquito caused infection.

    b. Determine vectorial capacity.

    c. Conduct laboratory tests of varying periods in which an *Ae. albopictus* mosquito feeds upon an infected animal and then is allowed to feed upon uninfected animals to see how many become infected with Zika.

    d. Assess mortality rate of infected *Ae. albopictus* in laboratory experiments.

Answer: a. Testing those infected with Zika to determine the species of mosquito is not feasible. However, assessing vectorial capacity and conducting lab experiments will result in better understanding. **Vectorial capacity** is the metric that will determine if *Ae. albopictus* is capable of serving as an efficient vector for Zika. The first parameter that one would want to know is if *Ae. albopictus* is a competent vector for Zika. In other words, can Zika multiply in *Ae. albopictus* to a level that would make it efficiently transmitted by this mosquito? This question can be answered with laboratory infection studies. One can infect an animal model with Zika and allow *Ae. albopictus* to feed upon the infected animal. You could then hold the fed mosquitoes in the laboratory for varying periods of time and then allow them to feed upon uninfected animals and see how many of the uninfected animals become infected with Zika. While conducting these laboratory studies, you could also measure the mortality rate in the infected mosquitoes and thus estimate the daily survival probability. Finally, by allowing the infected mosquitoes to feed upon susceptible animals at several different time points following their initial exposure to Zika, one could get an estimate of the extrinsic incubation time. These laboratory studies will give you estimates of three of the five parameters that you will need to estimate vectorial capacity. For the other two parameters, density and feeding preference, it will be necessary to conduct field studies. You can start by setting up traps and collecting mosquitoes to see how common *Ae. albopictus* is, both in absolute terms and relative to the other mosquito species found in your area. Finally, you can collect blood-fed mosquitoes from your field sites and identify the hosts that *Ae. albopictus* is feeding on in your area. This will provide you with all the information you need to determine if *Ae. albopictus* is likely to be a successful vector for Zika virus.

2. Models of Ebola virus transmission have demonstrated that the most important drivers in maintaining viral transmission are person-to-person contact with ill individuals or contact with the bodies of individuals who have died as a result of the disease. Which of the following would NOT be an effective intervention plan to stop an Ebola epidemic?

    a. Public education campaigns can be used to inform the population of the ways the virus is transmitted and encourage them to reduce contact with bodies of persons who have died.

    b. Making personal protective equipment (gloves, disposable gowns, surgical masks, etc.) widely available to the population, allowing home caregivers to protect themselves.

c. Requiring the immediate burning of all deceased bodies infected with Ebola.

d. Encouraging individuals who are feeling sick to self-report to health care facilities that have the capability of providing effective infection control measures.

Answer: c. The model suggests that minimizing contact between well and infected individuals or the bodies of individuals who have died from Ebola is the best way to stop the epidemic. There are several ways one might consider trying to minimize such contacts. However, forcing a community to burn or dispose of bodies without regard to local customs and practices is not an effective approach.

3. Blood lead levels are an agent of great concern with respect to public health and specifically children. Until 2012, children were identified as having a blood lead "level of concern" if the test result was 10 or more micrograms of lead per deciliter of blood. CDC is no longer using the term "level of concern" and is instead using the reference value to identify children who have been exposed to lead and who require case management. In the past, blood lead level tests below 10 micrograms per deciliter of lead in blood may, or may not, have been reported to parents.

Experts now use a reference level of 5 micrograms per deciliter to identify children with blood lead levels that are much higher than most children's levels. This new level is based on the US population of children aged 1 to 5 years who are in the highest 2.5% of children when tested for lead in their blood. This reference value is based on the 97.5th percentile of the National Health and Nutrition Examination Survey's (NHANES's) blood lead distribution in children. NHANES is a population-based survey to assess the health and nutritional status of adults and children in the United States and determine the prevalence of major diseases and risk factors for disease. The new lower value means that more children will likely be identified as having lead exposure allowing parents, doctors, public health officials, and communities to take action earlier to reduce the child's future exposure to lead.

Which of the following is this an example of?

a. How evidence-based biological claims can influence legislation enacted to protect the health of the public

b. How children remain the most vulnerable in our society

c. An overcautious approach

d. How political agendas can influence legislation

Answer: a. The issue of lead is a clear example of how public health researchers are using evidence-based biological claims to influence legislation that has been enacted to protect the health of the public. The other answers are not supported by the information.

4. Over the past 30 years, the effects of lead have been well studied experimentally including epidemiologic studies. Biologically based studies involving the absorption, distribution, metabolism, elimination, and storage of lead are well known. It is further recognized that the developing fetus and children with developing nervous systems are especially vulnerable to

lead toxicity. The sources of lead, especially for children, have become an issue of major concern. Which of the following is the most common route of exposure for children?

a. Old toys
b. Old paint
c. Contaminated soil
d. Unsanitary water

Answer: b. Lead-based paints are an important source of elevated blood lead levels in children. Homes built before 1978, when federal regulations changed, may still contain lead-based paints. Although lead can affect anyone, children are at highest risk, especially small children, who may put things in their mouths. The other mechanisms are not the best choices for the answer.

5. Which of the following is the leading cause of death in children in the United States?

a. Opioids and poisonings
b. Motor vehicle injuries
c. Burns
d. Suicides

Answer: b. While opioids have emerged as a serious injury problem within adults, the leading cause of death remains motor vehicle injuries for children. The other causes of injury death, although they are important, are not the leading cause of death for children.

6. Which of the following diseases may occur when pregnant women come into contact with infected cat feces?

a. Rubella
b. Toxoplasmosis
c. Down's syndrome
d. Phocomelia

Answer: b. Toxoplasmosis is a disease that results from infection with the *Toxoplasma gondii* parasite; infection is linked to undercooked contaminated meat, exposure to infected cat feces, and mother-to-child transmission. The other diseases or syndromes do not develop from infected cat feces.

7. There are many chemical agents that can cause diseases or disorders in humans. Which of the following would public health professionals suspect if a patient had symptoms of muscle spasms, nausea, vomiting, and abdominal pain? Another clue is that the product that is suspected to carry the agent is fertilizer.

a. Arsenic
b. Mercury
c. Asbestos
d. Organic solvents.

Answer: a. These symptoms and sources are characteristic of arsenic and not the others.

8. Susie is a environmental health specialist and has just received information from her supervisor that she needs to do a risk assessment for a new chemical agent found in laundry detergents. Which of the following should Susie embark on first as she implements this task?
   a. Determination of the LD_{50} of the chemical
   b. Peformance of a dose–response relationship
   c. Characterizing the risk for humans
   d. Performing a hazard assessment

Answer: The best response to this question is d., performing a hazard assessment. This is the first step of a risk assessment to determine if the chemical under consideration is likely to cause disease in humans. The other choices refer to procedures done after a hazard assessment to further assess the risk.

9. The most common route of exposure to chemicals in the human body is:
   a. Orally
   b. Inhalation
   c. Dermally
   d. Ingestion

The correct answer is b. Other choices are not the most common route.

10. Eutrophication of a waterway can be initiated when which of the following enters a lake or stream?
   a. Chloramines
   b. Synthetic organic chemicals
   c. Phosphates
   d. Volatile organic compounds (VOCs)

Answer: c. Eutrophication occurs when a body of water becomes overenriched with minerals and nutrients, resulting in excessive plant and algael growth or "bloom." This almost always occurs as a result of nitrate- or phosphate-containing detergents, fertilizers, or sewage making their way into the water. Based on the preceding information, b is not correct. Chloramines are added to the water to disinfect. VOCs are organic compounds that easily become vapors and thus would not end up in the water stream.

11. Which of the following are not greenhouse gases?
   a. Carbon dioxide and methane
   b. Nitrogen and oxygen
   c. Nitrous oxide and chlorofluorocarbons
   d. Water vapor and ozone

Answer: b. The primary greenhouse gases in the earth's atmosphere are water vapor, carbon dioxide, methane, nitrous oxide, and ozone. Chlorofluorocarbons and hydrofluorocarbons are also greenhouse gases. Nitrogen and oxygen are not considered greenhouse gases.

12. Biochemical oxygen demand (BOD) indicates the following:
   a. The potential amount of oxygen that the sample could contain given the pH, temperature, and volume
   b. The rate at which oxygen is being consumed by microorganisms living in the water
   c. The rate at which oxygen is produced
   d. The level of pollution

Answer: b. BOD is the measure of the quantity of oxygen used by aerobic bacteria and other microorganisms in the oxidation of organic matter.

13. Lethal dose (LD_{50}) values are determined by the amount of a substance that does the following:
   a. Kills those exposed to 50 grams of the substance
   b. Kills at least 50 individuals exposed to the substance
   c. Kills a population when given at least 50 milliliters of the substance
   d. Kills 50% of those exposed to the substance

Answer: d. LD_{50} is determined by the dose at which 50% of the exposed population will die. Other responses are not correct.

14. Which of the following is NOT a criteria air pollutant?
   a. Nitrogen
   b. Ozone
   c. Carbon monoxide
   d. Particulate matter

Answer: a. The Clean Air Act requires EPA to set NAAQS for carbon monoxide, lead, ground-level ozone, nitrogen dioxide, particulate matter, and sulfur dioxide. These are also known as criteria air pollutants.

15. Which of the following is NOT true about the herd immunity threshold?
   a. The threshold is NOT associated with the effectiveness of a vaccine.
   b. The threshold depends upon how easily a disease is transmitted.
   c. The herd immunity threshold for measles in a population is 95%.
   d. The herd immunity threshold for polio in a population is between 80% and 85%.

Answer: a. Herd immunity is a means of protecting a community by immunizing a critical mass. The threshold relates to how much of the population must be vaccinated to ensure herd immunity. Thus, the threshold is directly related to vaccine use and effectiveness. In addition, the threshold is dependent, in part, on how easily a disease is transmitted. Thus, different diseases have different thresholds. For diseases that are extremely contagious such as measles, a high immunity threshold (95%) is required to protect the populace. For other diseases that are a little less contagious, the threshold is slightly lower, 80% to 85%.

CONCLUSION

This chapter summarized the public health focus on biological determinants of health and reviewed emerging and reemerging infectious disease, noncommunicable and chronic diseases, and the biological determinants of health. In addition, this chapter covered the biological concepts that help to influence environmental laws and policies. The diseases and conditions referenced in this chapter will continue to plague populations globally, and it is imperative that we, as public health professionals, continue our efforts to assess these problems, understand the primary risk factors, and develop programs to prevent these conditions. The chapter also reviewed the factors that influence healthy environments, including those that adversely affect our air, land, and water.

REFERENCES

1. Aschengrau A, Seage GR. *Essentials of Epidemiology in Public Health.* 3rd ed. Burlington, MA: Jones & Bartlett Learning; 2013.

2. McDowell I. Epidemiologic triad. Available at: https://www.med.uottawa.ca/sim/data/Pub_Infectious_e.htm#epi_triad. Accessed June 26, 2018.

3. Battle CU. *Essentials of Public Health Biology: A Guide for the Study of Pathophysiology.* 1st ed. Sudbury, MA: Jones & Bartlett Publishers; 2009.

4. Muka T, Imo D, Jaspers L, et al. The global impact of non-communicable diseases on health-care spending and national income: a systematic review. *Eur J Epidemiol.* 2015;30(4): 251–277.

5. Moore GS. *Living With the Earth: Concepts in Environmental Health Science.* 3rd ed. Boca Raton, FL: Taylor & Francis Group; 2007.

6. World Health Organization. *Global Status Report on Noncommunicable Diseases 2014.* 2014. Available at: http://www.who.int/nmh/publications/ncd-status-report-2014/en. Accessed April 14, 2018.

7. Macdonald G. Epidemiological basis of malaria control. *Bull World Health Organ.* 1956;15(3): 613–626.

8. Bollyky TJ, Templin T, Cohen M, Dieleman JL. Lower-income countries that face the most rapid shift in noncommunicable disease burden are also the least prepared. *Health Aff (Millwood).* 2017;36(11):1866–1875.

9. Institute for Disease Modeling. SEIR and SEIRS models. Available at: http://idmod.org/docs/tuberculosis/model-seir.html. Accessed May 4, 2018.

10. Jones JH. Notes on R_0. Available at: https://web.stanford.edu/~jhj1/teachingdocs/Jones-on-R0.pdf. Accessed May 4, 2018.

11. Harris RE. *Epidemiology of Chronic Disease: Global Perspectives.* 1st ed. Burlington, MA: Jones & Bartlett Learning; 2013.

12. Prince MJ, Wu F, Guo Y, et al. The burden of disease in older people and implications for health policy and practice. *Lancet.* 2015;385(9967):549–562.

13. Xavier D, Pais P, Devereaux PJ, et al. Treatment and outcomes of acute coronary syndromes in India (CREATE): a prospective analysis of registry data. *Lancet.* 2008;371(9622): 1435–1442.

14. Feigin VL, Norrving B, George MG, Foltz JL, Roth GA, Mensah GA. Prevention of stroke: a strategic global imperative. *Nat Rev Neurol.* 2016;12(9):501–512.

15. Lozano R, Naghavi M, Foreman K, et al. Global and regional mortality from 235 causes of death for 20 age groups in 1990 and 2010: a systematic analysis for the Global Burden of Disease Study 2010. *Lancet.* 2012;380(9859):2095–2128.

16. Omran AR. The epidemiologic transition: a theory of the epidemiology of population change. *Milbank Q.* 1971;49(4):731–757.

17. McKeown RE. The epidemiologic transition: changing patterns of mortality and population dynamics. *Am J Lifestyle Med.* 2009;3(suppl 1):19S–26S.

18. Yusuf S, Reddy S, Ôunpuu S, Anand S. Global burden of cardiovascular diseases part I: general considerations, the epidemiologic transition, risk factors, and impact of urbanization. *Circulation.* 2001;104(22):2746–2753.

19. Reidpath DD, Allotey P. The burden is great and the money little: changing chronic disease management in low- and middle-income countries. *J Glob Health.* 2012;2(2):1–6.

20. Checkley W, Ghannem H, Irazol V, et al. Management of noncommunicable disease in low- and middle- income countries. *Glob Heart.* 2014;9(4):431–443.

21. World Health Organization. Global Action Plan for the Prevention and Control of NCDs 2013–2020. 2013. Available at: http://www.who.int/nmh/events/ncd_action_plan/en. Accessed April 14, 2018.

22. Watkins DA, Johnson CO, Colquhoun SM, et al. Global, regional, and national burden of rheumatic heart disease, 1990–2015. *N Engl J Med.* 2017;377(8):713–722.

23. Marijon E, Mirabel M, Celermajer DS, Jouven X. Rheumatic heart disease. *Lancet.* 2012;379(9819):953–964.

24. Centers for Disease Control and Prevention. Injury prevention & control. 2017. Available at: https://www.cdc.gov/injury/about/index.html. Accessed April 29, 2018.

25. Centers for Disease Control and Prevention. Opioid overdose. 2017. Available at: https://www.cdc.gov/drugoverdose/epidemic/index.html. Accessed April 29, 2018.

26. Glanz K, Rimer BK, Viswanath K. *Health Behavior: Theory, Research, and Practice.* 5th ed. San Francisco, CA: Jossey-Bass; 2015.

27. Friis FH. *Essentials of Environmental Health*. Sudbury, MA: Jones & Bartlett Publishers; 2007.

28. Centers for Disease Control and Prevention. Water treatment. 2015. Available at: https://www.cdc.gov/healthywater/drinking/public/water_treatment.html. Accessed April 29, 2018.

29. Doc Brown's Chemistry KS4 science GCSE/IGCSE/O Level Chemistry Revision Notes. Water cycle and water as a resource. Available at: http://www.docbrown.info/page01/AqueousChem/AqueousChem1.htm. Accessed May 5, 2018.

30. Malik O. Primary vs. secondary: types of wastewater treatment. Yale University. 2014. Available at: http://archive.epi.yale.edu/case-study/primary-vs-secondary-types-wastewater-treatment. Accessed April 17, 2018.

31. Centers for Disease Control and Prevention. Features of the RTECS Database. 2011. Available at: https://cdc.gov/niosh/rtecs/rtecsfeatures.html. Accessed April 29, 2018.

32. Farrell DJ, Bower L. Fatal water intoxication. *J Clin Pathol*. 2003;56(10):803–804.

33. World Health Organization. About us. Available at: http://www.who.int/about/en. Accessed May 4, 2018.

34. European Environment Agency. Available at: https://www.eea.europa.eu. Accessed April 29, 2018.

35. US Environmental Protection Agency. Available at: https://www.epa.gov. Accessed May 4, 2018.

36. Centers for Disease Control and Prevention. The National Institute for Occupational Safety and Health (NIOSH). Available at: https://www.cdc.gov/niosh/index.htm. Accessed May 4, 2018.

37. US Department of Labor. Occupational Safety and Health Administration. Available at: https://www.osha.gov. Accessed May 4, 2018.

38. Centers for Disease Control and Prevention. Agency for Toxic Substances and Disease Registry. Available at: https://www.atsdr.cdc.gov. Accessed May 4, 2018.

39. National Institute of Environmental Health Sciences. Available at: https://www.niehs.nih.gov. Accessed May 4, 2018.

6

Collaboration and Partnership

Jennifer Marshall, PhD, CPH, Pamela C. Birriel, PhD, MPH, CHES,
Rema Ramakrishnan, PhD, Dinorah Martinez Tyson, PhD, and
William M. Sappenfield, MD, MPH, CPH

INTRODUCTION

Developing effective partnerships and collaborations is essential to address the complex
public health issues that we face today. Key partners are needed to have the leadership,
expertise, resources, and reach to achieve a sustainable population-level impact. This
chapter will discuss the identification and recruitment of necessary stakeholders, assessment of the coalition's and team's capacity, establishment of an organizational framework,
development of operational plans and evaluations, and steps taken toward achieving sustainability. A short community example is provided to help with actualizing the process.
No matter your public health discipline, these concepts and skills are necessary for the
entire field of public health. The information presented focuses on collaboration and
partnership in public health practice and addresses the following tasks:

- ❏ Identify opportunities to partner with health and public health professionals across
  sectors and related disciplines.
- ❏ Identify key stakeholders.
- ❏ Identify critical stakeholders for the planning, implementation, and evaluation of
  health programs, policies, and interventions.
- ❏ Access the knowledge, skills, and abilities of health professionals to ensure that poli-
  cies, programs, and resources improve the public's health.
- ❏ Develop strategies for collaboration and partnership among diverse organizations to
  achieve common public health goals.
- ❏ Implement strategies for collaboration and partnership among diverse organizations
  to achieve common public health goals.
- ❏ Develop collaborative and partnership agreements with various stakeholders on specific projects.
- ❏ Manage partnerships with agencies within the national, state, or local levels of government that have authority over public health situations or with specific issues, such as
  emergency events.

❏ Apply relationship-building values and principles of team dynamics to plan strategies and deliver population health services.

❏ Develop procedures for managing health partnerships.

❏ Use knowledge of the role of public health and the roles of other health professions to appropriately address the health needs of individuals and populations.

❏ Establish roles, responsibilities, and action steps of key stakeholders in order to meet project goals and objectives.

❏ Engage key stakeholders in problem-solving and policy development.

❏ Implement methods of shared accountability and performance measurement with multiple organizations.

❏ Engage community partners in actions that promote a healthy environment and healthy behaviors.

MAJOR CONTENT

Building and Developing Partnerships

In the broadest sense, a partnership is a relationship in which two or more entities work together for a common purpose. These entities may be organizations, organizational systems, programs, community groups, or individuals operating at the local, regional, state, or national level. Partnership structures and processes vary widely (see Table 6-1). Collaborators may form a partnership agreement to work together in a cooperative or integrated relationship. Also, multiple individuals, groups, and organizations may come

Table 6-1. Definitions of Types of Partnership

Type of Partnership	Definition
Advisory board/committee	Advisory boards can serve multiple functions, such as informing the design, implementing and evaluating public health programs, identifying resources, reviewing policy, making recommendations, and providing input to decision-makers.
Task force	A task force is an action-oriented group that is tasked with addressing an issue or priority. The appointment of a task force may be time-limited. Members are brought together by an overseeing committee or institution.
Coalition	A coalition is a formal alliance of organizations that act jointly. They have a clearly defined leadership structure and may have shared or pooled resources. They can be time limited or sustained over a long period of time. Coalitions can be created at the community, state, regional, or national level.
Executive board/committee	An executive board is a formal group whose membership may be elected. It may provide oversight, strategy development, governing, and planning for a larger entity.

Source: Based on Butterfoss.[1]

together in a coalition or other structure to collectively impact communities. Partnerships are the bedrock of public health work to address the needs of communities.

How Is Community Defined?

Essentially, a community consists of a group of people who share a sense of collective identity, common values, goals, and institutions. Communities may be defined by geographic, administrative, cultural, or social boundaries.[2-4]

To effectively address complex public health issues, stakeholders from various sectors (e.g., health, policy, business, community, education, communications) and all levels of operation (e.g., community members, program participants/recipients, program implementers and designers, policymakers) within a societal system are needed. To collaborate is to work together toward a common vision and goal.[1] By aligning intentions and leveraging community resources, partners can improve community health and can also lessen the impact of health disparities.[5] Large-scale disasters such as floods, hurricanes, and bioterrorist attacks will also require collaboration among businesses, first responders, and other agencies to respond effectively. For example, in the aftermath of Hurricane Katrina, businesses provided essential resources to supplement government efforts, such as storage facilities, vehicles, and other needed supplies.[6]

Regardless of the structure and composition of the partnership, building and nurturing relationships will be the key to success and sustainability. It is critical to apply relationship-building values and principles of team dynamics to successfully plan strategies and deliver population health services. The Community Coalition Action Theory (CCAT) describes the structures and processes that encompass engagement and consensus-building efforts among diverse organizations and individuals to address community-level issues, recognizing the importance of leadership, membership, processes, structures, engagement, resources, assessment, and planning.[7] The stages of coalition development include **formation, maintenance,** and **institutionalization**. According to CCAT, communities can develop capacity to deal with problems and actively participate in making changes in the community. These changes, if self-developed and self-imposed, can lead to greater sustainability.[7-9]

Membership criteria should reflect the program goals, intended functions, and partnership purpose. Membership selection is an iterative process that entails identifying potential members and the best-suited engagement and recruitment strategies. Consider membership diversity, capacity, connections, expertise, knowledge, reputation, interest, personal agenda, and community ties and, where possible, build on existing relationships and organizational networks. It is also important to understand that a key informant(s) trusted by the community needs to be involved. Involving community members ensures that the problem you are trying to focus on has been identified and potentially owned by the affected community.

How Do You Identify Key Stakeholders?

When building and developing partnerships, you must first identify key **stakeholders** with whom to collaborate. When you get together for a mutually beneficial initiative, strategic relationships can develop with stakeholders.[7] Key stakeholders include individuals representing diverse organizations, factions, or constituencies within the community (e.g., community members, advocates, policymakers, researchers, service providers, administrators). These stakeholders agree to work together for the purpose of achieving a common goal.[7,9] Stakeholders may be any individuals interested or vested in the project or organization. **Gatekeepers** can be described as those who formally or informally control access to a priority population or control specific aspects of a community. **Opinion leaders** are respected community members who can represent the views of the priority population.[10]

Frequently, you may have a stakeholder workgroup consisting of 8 to 10 members. Sometimes you may select more if you are concerned about the level of people's participation. In the upcoming infant mortality case study, you will have the opportunity to consider a list of potential stakeholders. If you have trouble answering the case study questions, do not worry! There are many ways to identify and recruit key stakeholders. The stakeholder mapping exercise given in the Centers for Disease Control and Prevention's (CDC's) evaluation workbook can be a useful tool for this purpose.[11]

An overarching vision or goal is not enough to achieve success in addressing a complex public health issue. You will need to join with community partners to identify and prioritize needs, assets, and/or resources that can be used to address the issues. You want to define some common ground upon which you can work together collaboratively. It is important to think and plan ahead during this phase of collaboration so that you know what you want to do, who is on your side, who your opponents may be, and how to assess the problem you would like to solve. You may even want to define what the stages of success might look like. Conducting a needs assessment allows you to understand the issues, opposition, and community opinion (see Chapter 7, "Program Planning and Evaluation," for more information on needs assessments). With this information, identifying and selecting key stakeholders will enable the implementation of strategies for collaboration and partnership. In addition to formal roles in the community, the combined strengths, skills, and talents of these stakeholders contribute to the synergy. Sample questions for identifying key stakeholders are provided in Box 6-1. The process is iterative: partners are needed to conduct community assessments and the community assessment may identify additional partners.

Health professionals may have clinical expertise, as well as knowledge and experience with diverse individuals, health care management, and delivery systems. **Public health professionals** have the expertise to assess and address population- or community-level challenges and solutions, including the environmental and social determinants of health. As a public health professional, you have various skills and abilities that may

Box 6-1. Sample Questions You Can Ask Yourself to Help Find Common Ground and Identify Key Stakeholders

---

- What is the problem you are trying to address?
- Who are the key players and stakeholders related to addressing the problem?
- Who is affected by the issue or problem?
- What type of changes are needed (e.g., legislation, regulation, legal decision, committee action, institutional practice, or other)?
- Who is already working on this issue?
- Have you considered partnering or joining existing groups?
- What resources and/or assets can be built upon?
- What are the financial and political implications of the proposed change?
- What may be potential unintended consequences of working together?

Source: Based on Center for Community Health and Development at the University of Kansas.[12]

crosscut the different areas of public health. You may possess skills that are unique to your area of work. You may also be in various stages of your career. Some of you may be skilled at data analysis (qualitative or quantitative); others in communicating effectively. You may have experience in one or more of the following areas: advocacy, leadership, laboratory skills, management, development of software programs, or data visualization. To implement policies and programs, you need to collaborate despite your varied backgrounds, skills, and abilities. No one person can do everything effectively and efficiently in a timely manner. You need to be aware of evidence-based practices and programs and possess the ability to synthesize evidence. Public health training includes cultural competence and a fundamental understanding of health disparities, with a commitment to health equity—a perspective that is essential for success. (To learn more about health disparities, see Chapter 10.)

There are several ways that you can access knowledge, skills, and abilities. The most common and scholarly way to access these is to maintain continuing education credits by attending seminars and conferences to keep abreast of current developments in your field. A more active way to update your skills, learn how to solve a problem using new methods, or implement a new program is to attend training workshops, which are frequently offered at national meetings. For example, participating in a professional development training or a workshop may enable you to update your skills and learn about additional advancements in the field and emerging methods and technologies (e.g., how to calculate the cost-effectiveness of a program, how to utilize new technologies to enhance evaluation). One way to assess your knowledge and skills is to use online tools. These tools can identify gaps in your knowledge and provide information on how to improve your skills. Many state and national professional organizations offer these resources in conjunction with annual meetings or conferences, or as stand-alone institutes.

The Council on Linkages Between Academia and Public Health Practice has developed core competencies for three tiers of the public health professional in eight domains.[13]

These tiers reflect the career stages of the public health professional—tier 1: front-line staff or entry-level, tier 2: program management or supervisory level, and tier 3: senior management or executive level. The eight domains are (1) analytical/assessment, (2) policy development/program planning, (3) communication, (4) cultural competence, (5) community dimensions of practice, (6) public health science, (7) financial planning and management, and (8) leadership and systems thinking.

A self-assessment tool for each level of practice is publicly available. For each level, the assessment takes about 20 minutes to complete.[14–16] For those in the field of maternal and child health, another way to gain competence is to utilize online resources, such as the one provided by the MCH Navigator.[17] The MCH Navigator Web site provides excellent information on how to find learning opportunities in each of the domains.

To form partnerships, you may need key stakeholders drawn from members of the community who represent a diverse array of sectors and professional fields and have a variety of perspectives. They may need to be part of the previously mentioned knowledge, skills, and abilities assessment. Over the past three decades, the development of coalitions by community-based organizations to support health-related activities has increased. Members of advisory boards and/or coalitions may represent diverse stakeholders. To recruit community members, consider reaching out through community hubs—schools, churches, businesses, neighborhood associations—with careful consideration of the representativeness and diversity of those members.

You will develop relationships and partnerships with various stakeholders at the local, state, regional, and national level. Collaborative partnerships, guided by community organizing principles and processes, vary by level of commitment, activities undertaken, membership composition, and intensity (e.g., meeting frequency). Green and Kreuter defined these community organization principles and processes as the following:

> The set of procedures and processes by which a population and its institutions mobilize and coordinate resources to solve a mutual problem or to pursue mutual goals.[18]

Some contextual factors have an impact on the effectiveness of the collaboration, such as whether you should take into account the sociopolitical environment, trust between community sectors and partnering organizations, and community readiness.[7] Partnerships can also serve as a source of stability at times of organizational change.[19]

How do you build and maintain partnerships with agencies within the national, state, or local levels of government that have authority over public health situations or with specific issues, such as emergency events? Frequently your partnerships and coalitions may include, be funded by, or be led by governmental public health agencies. Public health agencies play an important and vital community role. They may have delegated authority (e.g., emergency response), designated funding (e.g., Zika grant funding), or identified the issue as a public health priority (e.g., opioid epidemic). In many situations, these agencies are valuable and essential partners for success. Besides funding, these agencies can provide other necessary resources (e.g., data, expertise, or policy, legal, or regulatory guidance), connect you to a larger network of other expertise and resources, provide regulatory authority, or start the process to move toward policy and/ or regulatory solutions. Learning about their role, capacity, and political context related to the particular issue should be considered as part of your community and capacity assessments. As with any of the collaborating organizational partners, it will be important to know what the organization wants and requires. You will want to be familiar with their operational context, structure, and processes.

Ways to develop and implement strategies for collaboration and partnership include the following:

- Having a shared, mutually agreed upon vision;
- Determining the best strategy/approach;
- Including multiple perspectives;
- Delineating roles and responsibilities;
- Having collaborative and partnership agreement with various stakeholders on specific projects;
- Maintaining open and clear communication; and
- Relying on collaborative and transformational leadership.

Further details regarding each one are described in the paragraphs that follow.

Have a Shared, Mutually Agreed Upon Vision

A clearly defined, shared vision for success will be the guiding star for any partnership. That vision can be a broad vision statement, such as "Improve infant health in our county," or a specific, measurable goal, such as "Reduce infant mortality health disparities in our county by 20%." Clear vision, goals, and strategies need to be developed to define the partnership. The goals and objectives that are important to each stakeholder must be clarified so that duplication of efforts is minimized. Also, you must determine what they need from you. You will find the need to return to these collaboration pillars over time to ensure alignment or you may need to adjust accordingly. The Community Toolbox offers several tips on creating a vision and building consensus among stakeholders.[12,20] There are group facilitation methods—such as paired listening, story boarding, nominal group technique, and ranking—that help to generate discussion and establish a unified vision (see Chapter 7, "Program Planning and Evaluation," for more information on shared vision).[21]

Determine the Best Strategy/Approach

Once that vision is established, the group needs to determine what would be the best strategy or strategies for reaching that goal. Deciding on the appropriate strategy or strategies is not easy—the group will need to review what has been tried before, what has been successful elsewhere, or, for similar issues, whether there are evidence-based or informed programs to replicate or adapt what is feasible and especially what is the best fit for the community.

Each stakeholder will have a specific viewpoint, set of priorities, knowledge and skills, and agenda. You may find that the best solution to a problem is not implementation of a new program but rather better coordination among existing programs, system changes to improve access and effectiveness of programs and to address gaps or bottlenecks in services, or a policy change. Policy development is the process of drafting new policies or revising existing policies. Policy development entails "conducting policy-relevant research, communicating findings in a manner that facilitates action, developing part-nerships, and encouraging the efficient use of resources through the promotion of poli-cies based on science—such as the promotion of evidence-based health interventions."[22] Policy advocacy includes the actions of a group to raise awareness or influence public opinion for or against policies or proposed policy changes.[23] This can be done via media campaigns or public service announcements, official proclamations, public demonstra-tions or other highly visible events, or disseminating information throughout various communication channels (e.g., publications, presentations, or online). If the expertise is not already at the table, additional partners may be engaged.

Include Multiple Perspectives

A critical component of building strong collaborations is to bring together and involve multiple stakeholders, as well as the communities that are affected by the problem and/ or have the resources to address them. Once the strategies for collaboration are devel-oped, external factors such as the right timing, the issue at hand, and the social target are critical for success in implementation.[24] Successful collaborations are made up of interde-pendent stakeholders; have a constructive way to deal with differences and or conflicts; share decision-making and power; have expectations and responsibilities clearly defined and mutually agreed upon, through either formal or informal agreements; and acknowl-edge that the process is fluid and dynamic.[25] Successful partnerships engage in brain-storming techniques—where all ideas are welcome and discussed. If partners can be open to the unexpected and share ideas freely, it will create an environment that encour-ages openness, innovation, and thinking outside the box.

Delineate Roles and Responsibilities

Outlining roles and responsibilities will help group members move effectively toward achieving common goals. One way to examine roles and responsibilities of stakeholders is to categorize stakeholder engagement in action into four levels: inform, consult, involve, and collaborate/empower. This is based on a report developed by the Los Angeles Department of Children and Family Services.[26] It describes when each level is appropriate and when it is not. For example, the level "involve" indicates that stakeholders are actively engaged in the project by providing input and participating in activities, but they do not make any decisions. In contrast, to "collaborate" implies equal power in the relationship.

Collaborative and Partnership Agreements With Various Stakeholders on Specific Projects

Collaborative agreements, such as a memorandum of agreement, provide documentation of the agreement and help to minimize potential disagreements, provide accountability, describe deliverables, and act as a reporting or dissemination mechanism. The agreements should include enough detail to guide the partnership and serve as a mechanism through which partners can assess the fulfillment of their commitments.[27] You should recognize that partners may need to consult with their legal or financial advisors before finalizing an agreement and this may take some time. Several meetings may be needed to develop an agreement that reflects everyone's needs and capacity. You may also need to select and use a collaborative planning process. Potential processes are discussed later in this chapter.

Maintain Open and Clear Communication

You will need to have open and clear communication, as well as send regular updates on progress and outcomes. This includes active listening where you focus on not only what people say but also on the underlying meaning. Your responses reflect that you have listened and acknowledge what has been said. Active listening can enhance relationships across partnerships. This may also include developing joint reports to keep all stakeholders equally informed and engaged. Other communication strategies include updates during meetings, newsletters or briefs, online discussion boards, or other technological approaches. You need to move toward the concept of shared accountability and recognize effort and accomplishments. It is important to find ways to celebrate successes, as well as to acknowledge challenges to help keep the coalition engaged and energized.

Rely on Collaborative and Transformational Leadership

Effective partnerships are also supported by collaborative and transformational leadership (see Chapter 3, "Leadership," for more information on leadership styles and strategies). Leadership within partnering community organizations supports buy-in and facilitates participation and implementation. Leadership across multiagency partnerships supports many functions of collaborative work. Hence, a key component of the Collective Impact Framework is the backbone organization, which performs functions that include guiding the overall vision and strategy, supporting aligned activities, establishing shared measurement practices, building public will, advancing policy, and mobilizing funding.[28]

Mobilization and Achieving Outcomes

Once stakeholders have been identified and engaged, a blueprint needs to be established for the planning, implementation, and evaluation of the community health actions (programs, policies, or interventions). In developing this blueprint, there are a couple of ways to conceptualize community planning approaches to implementing health actions. In one approach, the collaborative effort is led by community members with the support of partners. Alternatively, the effort may be led by organizations in partnership with community members.

The first approach may entail **community development**, in which the community aims to develop group identity and cohesion to build consensus and capacity. Alternatively, it may entail **community organizing**, which focuses on the process by which community groups identify common problems and goals, mobilize resources, and identify ways to reach goals. Key concepts in community-led public health actions are found in Box 6-2.

There are several community planning approaches. If organizations are leading the effort, then social planning or social action models may be used. **Social planning** models stress problem-solving and usually rely on expert practitioners to solve problems. **Social action** approaches focus instead on an overarching goal to increase community capacity to solve problems and achieve concrete changes that address social injustices. Regardless of the approach, public health focuses on initiatives serving populations, not individuals.

A mobilization plan should include clearly outlined roles, responsibilities, and action steps of the stakeholders. How do you identify the role and responsibility of each stakeholder? Most importantly, why do you need to establish these roles and responsibilities? The answers to these questions overlap each other. Thoughts in the opposite direction are also important. Considerations beyond the overall community benefits, specific benefits, or return on investment to each partner should be assessed to help ensure engagement. Organizations may adopt different strategies for evaluating public health programs

Box 6-2. Key Concepts in Community-Led Public Health Actions

- **Empowerment:** Community members gain or expand their own power to create change.
- **Community capacity:** Community members gain skills, social networks, and access to power through their participation.
- **Participation:** Community members develop and contribute leadership skills, knowledge, and resources through their involvement in community change.
- **Relevance:** Community members create an agenda for change based on their perceived needs, available resources, and shared power.
- **Issue selection:** Community members participate in identifying issues; specific targets for change are chosen as part of a larger strategy.
- **Critical consciousness:** Community members discuss the root causes of problems and plan actions to address them.

Source: Based on Wallerstein et al.[29]

or interventions. With CDC's classic Framework for Evaluation in Public Health, you will find six steps for program evaluation; engaging stakeholders is one them. (See Chapter 7, "Program Planning and Evaluation," for more information.)[11,30]

As organizational and community member coalitions mobilize to address problems, several planning models can be useful in structuring steps. Using a planning model helps to ensure that no important components are missed. It verifies that everyone has the same understanding of the process and that the group has a way to monitor its progress. An example of a model is the predisposing, reinforcing, and enabling constructs in educational/ecological diagnosis and evaluation (PRECEDE)–policy, regulatory, and organizational constructs in educational and environmental development (PROCEED) planning model (see Chapter 7, "Program Planning and Evaluation," for more information on the PRECEDE–PROCEED model). Other models also have shared elements—assessment, issue selection, collaborative activities, measurement, and evaluation. Some of these models follow:

- **Community Coalition Action Theory (CCAT)**: Coalitions engage in core processes that include analyzing the problem, assessing needs and assets, action planning, implementing strategies, and monitoring outcomes.[7]
- **Collective Impact Framework**: Includes five conditions that have been shown to lead to success in collaborative efforts—a common agenda, shared measurement systems, mutually reinforcing activities, continuous communication, and backbone support organizations. This idea of "mutually reinforcing activities" described by Kania and Kramer emphasizes that diverse stakeholders working together will accomplish the most if each participant undertakes "the specific set of activities at which it excels in a way that supports and is coordinated with the actions of others . . . differentiated activities through a mutually reinforcing plan of action."[28] Thus, the activities fall within an overarching plan.[28]
- **The Planned Approach to Community Health (PATCH) Model**: Uses the broad participation of a wide spectrum of people at the local community level in goal determination and action. Community health problems are first prioritized, and then community members select the one to address. Phases in the process include community mobilization, data collection and organization, selection of health priorities, intervention plan development, and evaluation.[31]
- **Asset-Based Community Development (ABCD)**: In contrast to needs-based approaches, ABCD is a method that identifies and builds on the strengths and resources in a community, including human resources—the gifts, talents, and capacities of local citizens. The focus of ABCD is to mobilize community development through appreciative inquiry and collaborative action. Steps include mapping assets by conducting informal discussions and interviews (collecting stories), building relationships and organizing a core group of community leaders, mobilizing economic development and information sharing, convening the community (including broad

representation) to develop a shared vision and plan, mobilizing assets for community development, and leveraging outside resources (people, activities, investments) to support the asset-based and locally defined development efforts.[32]

- **Mobilizing for Action through Planning and Partnerships (MAPP)**: MAPP is a community-driven strategic planning process for improving community health. Facilitated by public health leaders, this framework helps communities apply strategic thinking to prioritize public health issues and identify resources to address them. MAPP is not an agency-focused assessment process; rather, it is an interactive process that can improve the efficiency, effectiveness, and ultimately the performance of local public health systems. Steps include organizing, visioning, assessments, strategic issues, goals/strategies, and action cycle. The first three involve organization of the group, creating a vision, and reviewing assessments that incorporate community themes and strengths of the local public health system, community health, and forces of change. From these steps, strategic issues are identified, then goals and strategies, and finally the action cycle linking planning, implementation, and evaluation.[33]

As collaborators move forward with implementing changes, you will need a system of **shared accountability and performance measurements**. It is a good idea for the group to identify milestones along the way—short-term and long-term goals help the group to continue to build on successes and maintain momentum and will indicate if the strategies seem to be working. This can be accomplished through creating logic models and using planning frameworks (see Chapter 7, "Program Planning and Evaluation," for more information on logic models and planning frameworks).

Engaging a group of key stakeholders is essential for timely implementation of programs or interventions. According to the CDC's Framework, one must be transparent about the evaluation plan so that any misunderstandings, hidden agendas, and competing interests are out in the open.[11,30] Planning is the key. The simple yet informative type of logic model can be used to put this information on the table. The Evaluation Plan Methods Grid is a useful tool to delineate roles and responsibilities of stakeholders along with shared understanding of the evaluation plan.[11,30] For example, if the evaluation question is to compare program effectiveness in reduction of unsafe sleep environments among newborn babies, then one can list the information in the grid (see Table 6-2).

Table 6-2. Example of an Evaluation Plan Methods Grid

Evaluation Question	Indicator/Performance Measure	Method	Data Source	Frequency	Responsibility
Compare program effectiveness to reduce unsafe sleep environment among newborn babies	Percentage of families who receive safe sleep education at home	Cross-sectional study	Surveys	Before and after funding period	Home visiting staff

How do you implement methods of shared accountability and performance measurement with multiple organizations? Is it possible to have a collaborative or community partnership if only a single organization is made accountable for achieving the goals and objectives? The answer to those questions is probably no. According to the Collective Impact Framework, public health problems cannot be solved in isolation. Multiple entities need to have a shared agenda to achieve a common goal and ensure shared measurement for joint accountability.[28] Although a backbone organization may coordinate the various collaborators involved in an initiative, no single organization can be responsible for the working of all activities.

For this purpose, one needs to implement some method(s) for shared accountability through aligning goals and performance measurements. For example, consider the case study given later in this chapter. Just as logic models can be used for establishing roles and responsibilities of stakeholders, they can also be used for measuring performance and listing shared accountability. As you go through a logic model, you can examine the inputs and activities listed and assess the activities or tasks that have been achieved and the progress made on each of them. Depending on the program stage of development, you can also re-examine the outputs and outcomes and see where they are with respect to program goals and objectives.

Did the project achieve its goals and objectives? You can do a process evaluation to examine if the activities are being carried out as planned. Some of the questions that you may ask are the following: Are there any parts in the project that are problematic and need attention? Are there enough people at appropriate levels doing their allocated work? Are training and finances properly allocated?

Performance measurement gives you an opportunity to assess the types and levels of contribution of each organization in the collaboration. These measurements of contribution can include each organization's contribution of time, staff, leadership roles, services, referrals, funding, etc. These measures can also be linked to each entity's roles and responsibilities that may help to avoid the "blame game" in the event of failure. Performance measurement can be a means to achieve quality improvement and track progress. Rather than focusing on others' shortcomings, it helps answer the question— what works?[34]

For performance measurement, it is beneficial to have a mission for the project and set **specific, measurable, achievable, relevant, and time-oriented (SMART) objectives** for each organization. You must relate performance measurement to goals and objectives. How each organization performs is primarily measured through quantitative measures from available data. A value matrix may be a useful way to assess the capacities and activities deemed important by stakeholders.[34] Through strong organizational support, joint accountability, and shared measurement, a collaboration can create a transparent environment resulting in better project management and success in achieving the goals and objectives.

PRACTICE QUESTIONS

See if you can answer the following questions about engaging community partners in actions that promote a healthy environment and healthy behaviors:

1. As a partnering organization, you can achieve your goals and objectives by engaging in continuous communication with community partners.[28] Community engagement can be defined as the "process of working collaboratively with and through groups of people affiliated by geographic proximity, special interest, or similar situations to address issues affecting the wellbeing of people."[30] Given this definition, at what stage of the project do you think you should first engage citizens from the priority population?
   a. Convening
   b. Planning
   c. Implementation
   d. Evaluation

Answer: a. Convening. If you thought you needed to involve community partners only during the planning stage and then at the end of the project, then you must return to your logic model and examine the questions, when and why. The most effective way to engage community partners is to involve them in all stages, including the early convening process.

The steps of evaluation can serve as a guide to engage community partners in all of these stages. These steps are not necessarily clearly demarcated, as the initial phase of an evaluation includes engaging stakeholders.[11,30] Community partners can be an integral component of each of these steps. During the planning stage, if they are involved in formulating the goals and objectives of the project, they are more likely to be vested in the execution. During the implementation phase, one of the ways to engage community partners in action is to identify their assets and resources. This may enable taking actions for long-term collaborations. Along the lines of ABCD, you can analyze each community partner's history of success in their community, recognize the importance of social capital, focus on a participatory approach to promote a healthy environment and healthy behaviors, and determine how local resources can be used for economic development.[35] In this way, not only are the community partners actively engaged in the process of improving public health, but also resources and leadership for the project are shared, which can promote sustainability. During the evaluation phase, community partners can help to focus on the evaluation design, gather credible evidence, and disseminate results to the community.

2. Community-based interventions employ strategies at multiple levels of the ecological model, with the understanding that each level is part of an embedded system and interventions that occur at one level can produce changes at other levels.
   a. True
   b. False

Answer: a. The correct response is true as interventions and evaluations focused on the socioecological model include a more complete understanding of the public health issue and interrelationships between multiple levels of the model.

Now that you have reviewed how to build, develop, and mobilize partnerships and to work toward achieving shared outcomes and develop strategies to measure progress, let us put this information together to see how it is illustrated in a case example of a community collaboration that is in place today.

The following example of an infant mortality workgroup that was developed as part of the statewide Florida Healthy Babies Initiative demonstrates partnership formation from the initial meeting throughout development and action planning to achieve the intended goal of reducing disparities in infant mortality rates in a county[36]:

In May 2016, in response to a call from Florida's Surgeon General to mobilize communities around infant mortality, a county health department examined its infant mortality rates, trends, disparities, and risk factors and then organized its first community meeting for the Florida Healthy Babies Initiative project. The state Department of Health required county health departments to convene partners and set SMART goals for year 1, year 2, and year 5 of this initiative with quarterly reporting of their progress the first year and annually thereafter. The health department in this case study partnered with two public health researchers from a nearby university to present the county's infant mortality statistics, then led an interactive discussion with community stakeholders on possible causes and solutions.

3. Who are potential stakeholders in the county that should be included?

Possible answers: Health department staff, nurses, physicians, real estate agents, police, firefighters, social workers.

The topics presented at the meeting included overall mortality rates, rates by primary causes of death, maternal and infant factors affecting infant health, and community-level factors that may affect infant mortality rates in the county. Also discussed were the county's strengths and challenges for addressing infant mortality. The meeting concluded with the attendees sharing their primary concerns and an invitation to community members to collaboratively chart a course of action to address disparities in infant mortality and reduce the rates in the county.

4. What strategies were used to create a collective vision for addressing infant mortality in this county?

Possible answers: Convening diverse stakeholders, sharing data, leading a discussion, and soliciting stakeholder input in formulating the goals and objectives of the project.

Following this community meeting, stakeholders were invited to reconvene for a series of planning meetings. An administrative assistant from the health department scheduled meetings regularly at a convenient time and location for stakeholders, sent consistent reminders before meetings, and sent minutes with action steps following each meeting. New partners were continually invited to participate in the collaborative, expanding and strengthening the network of partners. In subsequent meetings, five specific objectives were formulated, leading to an ongoing community partnership to address the health of pregnant women and babies in their county: (1) promotion of safe infant sleep practices, (2) promotion of breast-feeding, (3) reduction in substance abuse, (4) implementation of the Baby Friendly Hospital Initiative in at least one hospital, and (5) promotion of the use of the Edinburgh Postnatal Depression Scale tool. Also discussed were measurable indicators for each of the objectives. Once key stakeholders were identified, three workgroups were formed so that each of them could focus on specific activities: depression screening, safe sleep equipment, and safe sleep. It was also decided to support two existing workgroups in the county—the Breastfeeding Task Force and Substance Abuse Exposed Newborn Task Force.

5. How would you describe the role of the county Department of Health in the Healthy Babies Collaborative?

Possible answers: Convening organization, backbone organization, community leader.

6. What were some ways that the lead organization supported the collaborative partnership?

Possible answers: Infrastructure support, leadership, convened and recruited partners, mobilized collaborative through action planning, etc.

The strength of this coalition is the sustained enthusiasm of members; while new members and organizations continually join, many have been there since the beginning and continue to attend every meeting. The coalition uses meeting time for both large group discussions and as a time when the smaller workgroups get together to do their work. The meeting coordinators believe this structure has contributed to their success because members do not have to attend an additional meeting to do their work, making efficient use of time. Another strength is that members are respectful of each other and the networking that is taking place has increased understanding about services and goals between member agencies and organizations.

Active planning and implementation keep the group engaged, along with strategies to ensure accountability. Workgroups report to the larger group on their plans and progress, meeting minutes are distributed each month, and reports are submitted to the state agency. Financial support from the state Surgeon General aids the local coalition in implementing projects, such as giving safe sleep furnishings to those in need. The sustainability of this initiative is supported through consistent leadership and infrastructure to support monthly meetings, continuous community engagement and partnership, shared decision-making, and accountability. Celebrating successes is one way to energize a working group.

There have been several successes of this initiative. For example, a new partnership between the local methadone clinic and hospital was developed. This was done by the neonatal intensive care unit nurses who visit pregnant women quarterly at the methadone clinic to teach about what to expect from the hospital at the time of delivery, who now are teaching about safe sleep and other topics related to parenting.

Another success of the initiative is development of a community-wide process to identify parents in need of safe sleep furnishings, a fitted sheet, and educational packet and to make sure that all these items are accounted for as they get distributed. The coalition members also came to agreement on educational materials to use to educate the public on safe sleep so that messaging is consistent throughout the community. One partner agency (Healthy Families) agreed to help educate licensed home day care staff about safe sleep, and the local jail is interested in offering safe sleep education to inmates. Finally, one of the two local hospitals is participating in the "Baby Steps to Baby Friendly" initiative, which is a commitment and set of action steps toward achieving the World Health Organization's Ten Steps to Successful Breastfeeding in their hospital setting. While the coalition members have not developed a formal memorandum of understanding or utilized other accountability systems, they have developed informal explicit agreements on practices such as distribution of infant sleep furnishings, fitted sheets, and educational kits. Shared documents and distribution logs are also being developed.

7. What stage of MAPP represents the current activities of this collaborative?
   a. Organizing
   b. Visioning
   c. Assessments
   d. Goals/strategies
   e. Action cycle

Answer: e. Action cycle (final phase of MAPP) because the project has now linked the planning, implementation, and evaluation processes and is in operation.[33]

One of the challenges was that although it was decided to focus on baby boxes to promote safe infant sleep initially, some stakeholders were more in favor of portable cribs (e.g., Pack 'n Play) because of logistic and funding restrictions and concerns about the acceptability by families of baby boxes. The relationship building and culture of respect that has been established in the workgroup has helped to ensure that an open dialogue of various points of view is encouraged, allowing the workgroup members to actively discuss and weigh the information on safe sleep furnishing options in order to make the best decisions for their community and programs. This local Healthy Babies Initiative is still in existence 18 months after its inception, and the community members continue to meet monthly to discuss goals and objectives and the progress each workgroup has made so far.

8. What are some methods for evaluating this collaborative?

Possible answers: Stakeholder surveys, interviews, or focus groups to assess the collaboration processes. Also social network analysis can evaluate interagency collaboration. Performance outputs and outcome measures to assess the effectiveness of the collaborative on impacting short- and long-term goals should be developed.

CONCLUSION

This chapter described why effective and sustainable multisector and interdisciplinary partnerships and collaborations are essential to addressing complex public health challenges. Partnership types, structures, and processes were defined and presented, along with theoretical and community planning frameworks. These are useful in public health for planning, mobilizing, and evaluating partnerships and coalitions. The importance of relationship building was emphasized, and tips for identifying and engaging key stakeholders were shared. Strengths and needs assessments guide collaboration in developing priorities, and a shared vision along with specific and measurable action steps to attaining that vision provides a blueprint for action.

Because public health impacts require sustained efforts, maintaining strong and functional partnerships among diverse stakeholders, community members, and organizations is paramount. Several strategies for building and maintaining these partnerships were also outlined. The case study illustrated how careful planning at the local level, with support from state-level leadership, led to development of one county's Healthy Babies Initiative. Through strong leadership; attention to diverse, cross-sector, and mutually reinforcing relationships in the recruitment and engagement of partners; and provision of infrastructure support to maintain the ongoing collaborative processes, the initiative has demonstrated several successes. With the information and tools that public health has to offer, you can also be successful!

REFERENCES

1. Butterfoss FD. *Coalitions and Partnerships in Community Health*. San Francisco, CA: Jossey-Bass; 2007.

2. Allman D. Community centrality and social science research. *Anthropol Med*. 2015;22(3): 217–233.

3. Kelly K, Caputo T. *Community: A Contemporary Analysis of Policies, Programs, and Practices*. Toronto, ON: University of Toronto Press, 2011.

4. MacQueen KM, McLellan E, Metzger DS, et al. What is community? An evidence-based definition for participatory public health. *Am J Public Health*. 2001;91(12):1929–1938.

5. Salimi Y, Shahandeh K, Malekafzali H, et al. Is community-based participatory research (CBPR) useful? A systematic review on papers in a decade. *Int J Prev Med*. 2012;3(6):386–393.

6. Buehler JW, Whitney EA, Berkelman RL. Business and public health collaboration for emergency preparedness in Georgia: a case study. *BMC Public Health*. 2006;6(1):285.

7. Butterfoss FD, Kegler MC. The Community Coalition Action Theory. In: DiClemente RJ, Crosby RA, Kegler M, eds. *Emerging Theories in Health Promotion Practice and Research*. 2nd ed. San Francisco, CA: Jossey-Bass; 2009:238–276.

8. Bartholomew Eldredge LK, Markham CM, Ruiter RAC, Kok G, Parcel GS. *Planning Health Promotion Programs: An Intervention Mapping Approach.* 4th ed. San Francisco, CA: Jossey-Bass; 2016.

9. Feighery E, Rogers T. *Building and Maintaining Effective Coalitions. Guide No. 12. How-To Guides on Community Health Promotion.* Palo Alto, CA: Stanford Health Promotion Resource Center; 1989.

10. McKenzie JF, Neiger BL, Smeltzer JL. *Planning, Implementing, and Evaluating Health Promotion Programs: A Primer.* 4th ed. San Francisco, CA: Benjamin Cummings; 2005.

11. National Center for Chronic Disease Prevention and Health Promotion. Developing an Effective Evaluation Plan: Setting the Course for Effective Program Evaluation. Centers for Disease Control and Prevention. 2011. Available at: https://www.cdc.gov/obesity/downloads/cdc-evaluation-workbook-508.pdf. Accessed June 15, 2018.

12. Center for Community Health and Development at the University of Kansas. Community Tool Box. Available at: http://ctb.ku.edu/en/dothework/tools_tk_1.aspx. Accessed April 15, 2018.

13. Public Health Foundation. About the Core Competencies for Public Health Professionals. Available at: http://www.phf.org/programs/corecompetencies/Pages/About_the_Core_Competencies_for_Public_Health_Professionals.aspx. Accessed August 5, 2017.

14. Public Health Foundation. Competency assessment for tier 1 public health professionals. 2014. Available at: http://www.phf.org/resourcestools/Documents/Competency_Assessment_Tier1_2014.pdf. Accessed August 5, 2017.

15. Public Health Foundation. Competency assessment for tier 2 public health professionals. 2014. Available at: http://www.phf.org/resourcestools/Documents/Competency_Assessment_Tier2_2014.pdf. Accessed August 5, 2017.

16. Public Health Foundation. Competency assessment for tier 3 public health professionals. 2014. Available at: http://www.phf.org/resourcestools/Documents/Competency_Assessment_Tier3_2014.pdf. Accessed August 5, 2017.

17. National Center for Education in Maternal and Child Health. Self-assessment. Available at: https://www.mchnavigator.org/assessment. Accessed August 5, 2017.

18. Wildridge V, Childs S, Cawthra L, Madge B. How to create successful partnerships—a review of the literature. *Health Info Libr J.* 2004;21(suppl 1):3–19.

19. Green LW, Kreuter MW. *Health Program Planning: An Educational and Ecological Approach.* 4th ed. New York, NY: McGraw-Hill; 2005.

20. National Park Service. Rivers, trails, and conservation assistance program toolboxes. Available at: https://www.nps.gov/ncrc/programs/rtca/helpfultools/toolbox/dec_consensus.htm. Accessed April 15, 2018.

21. Seeds for Change. Facilitation tools for meetings and workshops. Available at: https://seedsforchange.org.uk/tools.pdf. Accessed April 15, 2018.

22. Centers for Disease Control and Prevention. Definition of policy. Available at: https://www.cdc.gov/policy/analysis/process/definition.html. Accessed April 15, 2018.

23. Cottrell RR, Girvan JT, McKenzie JF, Seabert D. *Principles and Foundations of Health Promotion and Education.* San Francisco, CA: Benjamin Cummings; 2002.

24. Mizrahi T, Rosenthal BB. Complexities of coalition building: leaders' successes, strategies, struggles, and solutions. *Soc Work.* 2001;46(1):63–78.

25. Gray B. *Collaborating: Finding Common Ground for Multiparty Problems.* 1st ed. San Francisco, CA: Jossey-Bass; 1989.

26. Western and Pacific Child Welfare Implementation Center, Los Angeles Department of Children and Family Services. Stakeholder engagement tools for action. 2013. Available at: https://www.cssp.org/publications/general/WPIC_DCFS_Stakeholder_Engagement_Toolkit.pdf. Accessed August 5, 2017.

27. John Snow. Engaging your community: a toolkit for partnership, collaboration, and action. Available at: http://www.jsi.com/JSIInternet/Inc/Common/_download_pub.cfm?id=14333&lid=3. Accessed April 15, 2018.

28. Kania J, Kramer M. Collective impact. *Stanford Soc Innov Rev.* 2011;9(1):36–41.

29. Wallerstein N, Minkler M, Carter-Edwards L, Avila M, Sanchez V. Improving health through community engagement, community organization, and community building. In: Glanz K, Rimer BK, Viswanath K, eds. *Health Behavior: Theory, Research, and Practice.* 5th ed. San Francisco, CA: Jossey-Bass; 2015:277–300.

30. McCloskey DJ, McDonald MA, Cook J, et al. Community engagement: definitions and organizing concepts from the literature. In: Centers for Disease Control and Prevention, ed. *Principles of Community Engagement.* 2nd ed. Bethesda, MD: National Institutes of Health; 2011.

31. Green LW, Kreuter MW. CDC's planned approach to community health as an application of PRECEDE and an inspiration for PROCEED. *J Health Educ.* 1992;23(3):140–147.

32. Kretzmann JP, McKnight JL. *Building Communities From the Inside Out: A Path Toward Finding and Mobilizing a Community's Assets.* Chicago, IL: ACTA Publications; 1993.

33. National Association of County & City Health Officials. MAPP Framework. Available at: http://www.naccho.org/topics/infrastructure/mapp/framework/index.cfm. Accessed April 15, 2018.

34. Lichiello P. *Guidebook for Performance Measurement.* 1999. Available at: http://www.phf.org/resourcestools/Documents/PMCguidebook.pdf. Accessed June 15, 2018.

35. Mathie A, Cunningham G. From clients to citizens: asset-based community development as a strategy for community-driven development. *Dev Pract.* 2003;13(5):474–486.

36. Florida Department of Health Office of Communications. Department invests $1.4 million in Florida Healthy Babies initiative. 2016. Available at: http://www.floridahealth.gov/newsroom/2016/03/031016-healthy-babies.html. Accessed June 15, 2018.

7

Program Planning and Evaluation

Karen D. Liller, PhD, CPH, Anna Torrens Armstrong, PhD, CPH, and Jennifer Marshall, PhD, CPH

INTRODUCTION

Program planning, implementation, and evaluation are instrumental to the work of many public health professionals. The information in this chapter will provide guidance on how to plan, implement, and evaluate successful public health programs. The chapter is divided into planning, implementing intervention, and evaluation components. A detailed case study follows that will allow you to apply much of what you learn in this chapter. The following tasks are focused on the domain of program planning and evaluation:

❑ Develop and conduct formative evaluation plans.
❑ Develop and conduct outcome evaluation plans.
❑ Develop process evaluation plans.
❑ Apply qualitative evaluation methods.
❑ Apply quantitative evaluation methods.
❑ Evaluate the benefits of qualitative or quantitative methods for use in evaluation.
❑ Assess evaluation reports in relation to their quality, utility, and impact.
❑ Assess program performance.
❑ Utilize evaluation results to strengthen and enhance activities and programs.
❑ Apply evidence-based practices to program planning, implementation, and evaluation.
❑ Identify challenges to program implementation.
❑ Ensure that program implementation occurs as intended.
❑ Plan evidence-based interventions to meet established program goals and objectives.
❑ Implement context-specific health interventions based upon situation analysis and organizational goals.
❑ Design context-specific health interventions based upon situation analysis and organizational goals.
❑ Plan and communicate steps and procedures for the planning, implementation, and evaluation of health programs, policies, and interventions.
❑ Design action plans for enhancing community or population-based health.
❑ Evaluate personnel and material resources.
❑ Use available evidence to inform effective teamwork and team-based practices.

❑ Prioritize individual, organizational, or community concerns and resources for health programs.

❑ Design public health interventions that incorporate such factors as gender, race, poverty, history, migration, or culture within public health systems.

❑ Develop a community health plan based on needs and resource assessments.

❑ Apply evaluation frameworks to measure the performance and impact of health programs, policies, and systems.

MAJOR CONTENT

Critical to the success of any planning model or framework is the garnering of support from those in positions to approve or make planning decisions and of course the community for whom the program is being planned. **Needs and resource assessments** are critical to the success of program planning efforts. A needs assessment is the process of identifying, analyzing, and prioritizing the needs of a priority population. Other terms that you may have heard of related to needs assessment are community analysis, community diagnosis, and community assessment.[1] In most cases, a planning process should begin with a thorough needs assessment. Needs assessments provide a logical place to start the process, help ensure the appropriate use of planning resources, identify important public health problems, determine the capacity of a community to address a specific need, and provide a focus for the development of a resulting intervention.[2] Sometimes a needs assessment is not needed. This may occur if there has already been one done recently, funding is available to address a specific issue, or the planner's employer has specified the need. For example, a health educator working in the cancer prevention section of a local agency would focus work on the cancer needs of the population.[1]

Stakeholder involvement and feedback are also vital. Stakeholders can assess the program and provide feedback throughout the planning and evaluation process. They are critical in the development of **vision, mission, objectives, strategies, and actions** (VMOSA). It is important to understand the differences among the vision, mission, goals, and values of the planning organization and resulting programs developed. According to the Community Tool Box, it is helpful to use VMOSA (http://ctb.ku.edu/en/table-of-contents/structure/strategic-planning/vmosa/main).[3] A **vision** communicates what your organization believes are the most ideal conditions for your community—the best it could be. These statements must be understood and shared by members of the community, and be broad, inspiring and uplifting, and easy to communicate. A vision might be a community free of colon cancer. The **mission** describes what the group is actually going to do and why. Mission statements are more concrete than vision statements. They should be one sentence, outcome-oriented, and inclusive. A mission statement related to the previous vision statement might be "Build primary and secondary prevention of colon cancer through comprehensive community and state health initiatives."

Table 7-1. Draft of Community Health Program Action Step

Step	Person Responsible	Date of Completion	Resources	Barriers or Resistance	Collaborators
Draft an education program on colon cancer	Sandy Jones from the planning committee and local university	January of next year	$1,500 for support of a student and meeting space and refreshments	None anticipated as long as planning group sees the value of this program	Members of the education subgroup, community health education programs

Objectives are much more specific than vision and mission statements. They should answer the questions of who, what, how much, and by when. These objectives can be behavior-, community-, and process-oriented, which is related to how the program will be implemented. Examples of objectives related to the colon cancer example are the following: sixty percent of the population aged 50 years and older (who and how much) will have a colonoscopy done (what) within 3 years of the program and repeated within a 10-year period (by when). A community objective might be that there will be a 50% increase in the number of health centers (who, what, and how much) that offer colonoscopy within 5 years of the program (by when). A process objective (related to activities) would be that 10 health educators will be hired by the health department (who and how much) to participate in the colon cancer prevention activities (what) three months before the start of the program (by when). SMART Objectives are specific, measurable, achievable, relevant, and time limited.

Strategies are how you will reach your objectives. These might include social marketing campaigns or community outreach activities. Lastly, an **action plan** is very helpful to spell out how a group will accomplish its objectives. Action steps are developed for every stage of the intervention. Components of the plan include the step (what will happen), person responsible (who will do what), date to be completed, resources required, barriers or resistance and how to overcome these, and collaborators. For example, if a step in an action plan is to develop a draft of a community health program on the risks for colon cancer, the example found in Table 7-1 could apply.

Program Development

Programs must have a rationale to be able to communicate with decision-makers, especially those decision-makers who are in charge of resources. In creating a rationale, program planners need to identify the health problem in global terms backed with data—and, if possible, what economic costs there are of the problem. Cost–benefit and return-on-investment findings are important here.

Next it is helpful to narrow the health problem by showing its relationship to a priority population. Proposed solutions to the problem need to be generated, and what will be gained from the program. Sources of information about the health topic and related public health programs can be found in a variety of sources, including the Community Tool Box and *The Guide to Community Preventive Services* (https://www.thecommunityguide.org), which summarizes the findings from systematic reviews of public health interventions.[4]

Your **planning committee** is critical to the success of your planning efforts. Who is on the committee is guided by the program, resources, and the situation at hand. Individuals to include are subgroups of the priority population to foster program ownership, someone with the health risk (if the program is focused on such a risk), people who care about the program and will do the tasks and have influence, someone who is a key leader in the organization that sponsors the program, and other related stakeholders. The key here is that everyone and anyone who has influence over or can contribute to the overall success of the program needs to be involved!

What Planning Model Should I Use?

There are many planning models to choose from in health promotion. Planning models have been defined as visual representations and descriptions of steps or phases in the planning process and are the means by which structure and organization are given to the successful development and delivery of health promotion programs.[2] While each model has some unique characteristics, it is helpful to think of all of them having all or nearly all the components of **The Generalized Model.**

This model encompasses the following steps:

1. Assessing need: On the basis of the collection and analysis of data, what are the health needs of your population? What are the priorities? Are there priority populations that need to be selected for the program?
2. Setting goals and objectives: What will happen? A goal is a broad statement of intent whereas objectives are more focused and answer questions such as who, what, how much, and by when—they are specific, measurable, action-oriented, relevant, and time limited or SMART.
3. Developing interventions: How will you meet your goals and objectives—is your intervention based on sound theory and logic?
4. Implementing interventions: How will you put your intervention into action?
5. Evaluating the results: What happened? Did the intervention meet its goals and objectives? How can you improve the quality of the program? Did you conduct formative and summative evaluations?[2]

Based on these steps, most planning models can be easily understood. Examples of planning models include the Centers for Disease Control and Prevention's (CDC's) **Planned Approach to Community Health (PATCH),** which was introduced in 1983 and used in partnership with state and local health departments and local communities. Its phases comprise the following:

1. Mobilizing the community
2. Collecting and organizing the data
3. Choosing health priorities and target groups
4. Choosing and conducting interventions
5. Evaluating the PATCH process and interventions[1]

Another planning model is **Assessment Protocol for Excellence in Public Health (APEX-PH)**, a project among several public health organizations including CDC, American Public Health Association (APHA), and National Association of County and City Health Officials (NACCHO). This planning model is used specifically for local health departments. There is also **Mobilizing for Action through Planning and Partnerships (MAPP)**. This model essentially replaced APEX-PH. Steps comprise the following:

1. Organizing for success and partnership development
2. Visioning
3. Four MAPP assessments
4. Identifying strategic issues
5. Formulating goals and strategies
6. An action cycle[1]

A new model, **MAP-IT**, was developed in 2010 to allow communities to implement their own adaptation of *Healthy People 2020*. The steps are mobilize, assess, plan, implement, and track.[1]

Two leading planning models used in health promotion are **predisposing, reinforcing, and enabling constructs in educational/ecological diagnosis and evaluation (PRECEDE)–policy, regulatory, and organizational constructs in educational and environmental development (PROCEED)** and **intervention mapping**.[5–7] The PRECEDE–PROCEED model has long been a planning model used in health promotion programs. It has gone through revisions and now encompasses eight steps that are the **social assessment,** which focuses on determination of **quality of life** of the population, then the **epidemiological assessment,** which encompasses the **health issue, and those behavioral, genetic, and environmental issues** related to each other and to the quality of life (phases 1 and 2, respectively). Then phase 3 is the **educational and ecological assessment** with the **predisposing, reinforcing, and enabling factors**. It is this phase in which the input of theory is quite important. Predisposing factors include knowledge and affective traits such as attitudes and beliefs that predispose one to change. Enabling factors are those resources and skills that are necessary for the behavior change. Also, there are barriers in these categories. The reinforcing factors involve feedback and reward systems that the program participants receive after the behavior change. Phase 4 is the **administrative**

and policy assessment and intervention alignment in which the health program is designed, and the educational strategies and administrative and policy factors need to be taken into consideration. Program budgets and resources are critical at this phase. Phase 5 is **implementation of the program** and **phases 6 through 8** focus on **program evaluation, from the most immediate or process evaluation to the farthest outcome evaluation.**[5]

To expand upon the intervention components, the **intervention mapping** model is quite helpful. This model has a series of steps with related matrices to guide the planner through the process. The steps comprise the following:

1. Developing a logic model of the health problem
2. Developing program outcomes and objectives with a logic model of change
3. Doing a program design
4. Producing the program
5. Developing a program implementation plan
6. Developing an evaluation plan[6]

The model developers suggest using PRECEDE as the framework for creating the logic model (theory) of the problem itself with graphic representations of the causal relations between health problems and their causes. The tasks relevant to creating a logic model of the problem include first establishing and working with a planning group; conducting a good needs assessment to create the logic model of the problem; describing a context for the intervention that includes the population, setting, and community; and then developing overall program goals. Also important to do is to develop the logic model of change by stating expected outcomes for the behavior and the environment, specifying performance objectives for behavioral and environmental outcomes, selecting determinants for the behavioral and environmental outcomes, constructing matrices of change objectives, and then creating the logic model for change with the preceding information. Change objectives are personal determinants × performance objectives. For example, if a performance objective is for the population to wear a bicycle helmet each time when riding a bike and a theoretical determinant is the need for self-efficacy, then a change objective could be that the target population expresses confidence in their ability to consistently use a helmet when riding a bike. Central to intervention mapping is the involvement of the community and planning group throughout—with much free-flowing brainstorming for each of the steps.[6]

Intervention Planning, Development, and Implementation

After goals, behavioral and environmental objectives, and the related change objectives are developed, the critical next step is to develop the set of activities that will constitute the intervention.[2] Planners go through several steps to ensure that the intervention is both effective and efficient in achieving the stated objectives.[2] The preferred approach is to identify intervention activities that already exist and are evidence-based to adopt or adapt, rather than designing a brand-new intervention. Developing a new intervention can be expensive and time and labor intensive. However, when evidence-based interventions are not available, this is also an option.

Adapting an Intervention

When adopting or adapting an intervention, we typically start by reviewing the existing evidence-based interventions. **Evidence-based** is an important concept in public health and public health interventions. We want both our goals and objectives to be evidence-based, meaning that they reflect current scientific evidence related to the behavior.[6] We also want to use evidence-based interventions, which commonly refers to those interventions that have been systematically developed using best practices in developing the intervention, as well as rigorously tested and shown to be effective in achieving the desired outcomes.[6]

There are many resources for identifying evidence-based interventions. A first step is to review the existing literature; however, the various resources available provide far more information than even a thorough literature review can offer. For example, CDC's *The Community Guide* (https://www.thecommunityguide.org) provides systematic reviews and recommendations on interventions and where they are with regard to **effectiveness (generalized results), efficiency (intervention-specific results),** and whether it is a recommended practice (or needs further testing).[4,6]

Other resources that can assist planners in identification of reviews of evidence-based interventions include the following:

- Agency for Healthcare Research and Quality Evidence-Based Practice Center Reports (https://www.ahrq.gov/research/findings/evidence-based-reports/index.html)[8]
- Canada's Health Evidence (https://www.healthevidence.org)[9]
- The Cochrane Collaboration Library (http://www.cochranelibrary.com)[10]

Access to full evidence-based interventions can be found at the following resources:

- US National Cancer Institute's Research-Tested Intervention Programs (http://rtips.cancer.gov)[11]
- US CDC's Effective Interventions: HIV Prevention that Works (https://effectiveinterventions.cdc.gov)[12]
- US Substance Abuse and Mental Health Services Administration National Registry of Evidence-Based Programs and Practices (http://www.samhsa.gov/nrepp)[13]

Once selected, an evidence-based intervention must be assessed for necessary changes to the intervention to increase fit for the given context. Program adaptation requires formative research to identify what elements must be adapted to the specific context and audience of your program. In the previously mentioned intervention mapping approach, Bartholomew Eldredge et al.[6] provide a set of steps for adapting and implementing evidence-based programs.

The first step includes a needs assessment, development of a logic model, a logic model of change, assessment of organizational capacity, and development of program goals. These steps have likely been performed. This is done in an effort to align the current program with existing evidence-based interventions. The second step involves searching for evidence-based interventions that are the best fit with the problem you are trying to address. The third step is a deeper look into fit, in which planners assess the need for potential adaptations needed including behavioral and environmental fit, determinants and change methods, delivery, design, and cultural fit, as well as implementation while determining if the core program elements can be retained. Rarely is a program adopted and replicated with no adaptation. Sometimes, the decision is that an evidence-based intervention is not available for replication or adaption. Then the planner should move on to intervention mapping program planning. However, if it is determined that adaptation is needed, the next step (step 4) is to make those changes, pretest related materials, and produce the final adapted materials. Step 5 includes developing a plan for implementation for the adapted program, and step 6 involves planning the evaluation.

Plan Evidence-Based Interventions to Meet Established Program Goals and Objectives

Should the decision be made that a new intervention be developed, it is a vital first step to consider existing evidence-based interventions and practices. While adoption or adaptation in full may not be practical or meet the needs of the priority population, reviewing the existing evidence-based interventions will provide insight into the appropriate strategy and methods that will be most successful for the intervention being developed.

Strategy is defined as a "general plan of action that may encompass several activities and considers the characteristics of the priority population."[14] The developed strategy helps shape the methods selected to meet the educational and environmental objectives.[14] Methods refers to the "systematic approach or procedures used by presenters, health educators or speakers to share information, objectives and lesson materials, and can also refer to a specific part of an intervention, lesson or presentation."[14] Method selection is critical in the transmission, reception, and retention of information by audiences.[14]

There are multiple intervention strategies that a planner might consider for the intervention. These can include health communication, health education, health policy, environmental change, health-related community service, and community mobilization, as well as others.[2] In exploring existing interventions, it is important to consider a variety of strategies, including local examples, examples from the professional literature, or national presentations. Brainstorming with the community, colleagues, and your community coalition can also generate ideas. The Community Tool Box (https://ctb.ku.edu/en) offers key questions to help decide on an intervention or parts of an intervention including the following[15]:

- Is it an appropriate fit for the group's purpose?
- Does the intervention strategy make a difference in behavior or outcome? (Is it effective?)
- Is there sufficient detail to replicate the intervention?
- Is it simple enough that people can do what is required?
- Do you have the resources (time, money, people)?
- Does it fit with local needs, resources, and values?

After considering these questions, as well as identifying potential barriers or resistance to a potential intervention, the key components of the intervention must be identified. Once these core components are selected, the methods to implement these strategies must be selected while taking into consideration the priority population, culture, and health literacy levels among other things (e.g., if sharing information is a core component, what method[s] can be used to share the information). Remember that selecting methods informed by theory and/or theoretical constructs will make a stronger intervention. It is also important to consider multiplicity and dose—the number of activities that make up the intervention and number of program units delivered, respectively.[2]

Bartholomew Eldredge et al.[6] provide a comprehensive review of theory-informed methods for changing behavior in a table format. Methods are presented by the targeted outcome—changing a determinant for at-risk individuals (e.g., attitudes, knowledge, awareness, risk perception) and changing determinants at various levels for the at-risk group, such as at social or physical levels.

The full tables are available in several online resources, including the following open-access publication in *Health Psychology Review*:

- Kok G, Gottlieb NH, Peters, GJ, et al. A taxonomy of behavior change methods; an intervention mapping approach. *Health Psychol Rev.* 2016;10(3):297–312.[16] (The tables are presented as a supplement to this article, but likewise can be accessed at the Open Science Framework [https://osf.io/sqtuz]).[17]
- A collection of resources on effective behavior change is available at https://effective behaviorchange.com.[18]

Pilot testing interventions can help save time and money and reduce the chance of program failure. Testing your intervention on a small scale allows for process evaluation and identification of unintended consequences, as well as the opportunity to incorporate critical feedback to improve and refine the intervention.

Identify Challenges to Program Implementation

Challenges to program implementation can often be reduced by ensuring ample consideration in advance during the planning stages. Challenges can include funding, fidelity of implementation, staffing issues, communication problems, and low participation. To identify (and anticipate) challenges to program implementation, including a formative evaluation and pilot implementation can be helpful steps. In addition, including a process evaluation, human resources management, and a monitoring plan will provide quick insight into emerging issues.

Ensure That Program Implementation Occurs as Intended (Fidelity of Implementation)

Training for program implementation and delivery is critical to implementation to ensure fidelity of implementation (the program is implemented as originally intended and according to the plan) as well as provide self-efficacy and morale for staff.[19] Program quality and fidelity can be managed by using a variety of strategies ranging from group development (for staff) and ongoing training to focusing on communication and program processes.[19]

Implement Context-Specific Health Interventions Based Upon Situation Analysis and Organizational Goals

Situation analysis refers to the consideration of community demographic, social, and economic parameters in any given community in conjunction with the highest-priority issues, goals, and resources of the planning committee.[5] It is an early critical step in which planner(s) "take stock" of the community and all of the related elements as planning begins to provide the needed context for planning.

A good starting place for situation analysis is the identification of stakeholders, potential collaborators, available staff and technical resources, and budget estimates.[5] Assessing community capacity and readiness, and engaging in **asset mapping** can help identify specific information related to the community context that will support the implementation of health interventions. Conducting a SWOT, or strengths, weaknesses, opportunities, and threats analysis, will help identify existing community strengths or assets that can support the intervention, identify weaknesses, and plan for opportunities and potential threats, which can be both internal and external.[20]

Evaluation of Programs

Quinn Patton describes evaluation as "the systematic collection of information about the activities, characteristics, and outcomes of programs, for use by people to reduce uncertainties, improve effectiveness, and make decisions."[21] According to CDC, evaluation can be approached as a systematic investigation of the merit, worth, or significance of a program.[22] Therefore, evaluation may serve a number of purposes. Outcome evaluation helps to determine the costs and benefits of a program and can be the basis for choices when resources are limited. Evaluation is also closely associated with identification of evidence-based best practices and with program improvement. Evaluation can be a source of information for improving programs and even policies because it leads to research questions that can be tested within a program or in other programs. Finally, public health agencies need to be accountable, and rigorous evaluation is increasingly mandated by funders and policymakers.

There are essentially three types of evaluation, **formative, process,** and **summative.** The type of evaluation to use depends on the stage of program development, resources available (time, personnel), and stakeholder needs. Formative evaluation assesses the context in which a program is developed and can include needs assessment or the development of components of a program. **Formative evaluation encompasses research conducted that contributes to the design of a program**. Needs assessment may identify and measure unmet needs within a community or assess the needs, priorities, and preferences of potential program participants. Program components or materials may be pilot-tested or adapted during this phase.

Process evaluation measures and describes the implementation of a program. Newer programs may not have been in place long enough to conduct summative evaluation. However, even for long-running programs, process evaluation is critical for understanding how and why a program works or does not work and can provide feedback on program implementation, content, methods, and participant, practitioner, and stakeholder response, particularly when adaptations have been made to the program design. Process evaluation is also helpful in describing how a program actually operates before offering the same services at additional locations or with other populations.

Two models are worth noting here. The first is **empowerment evaluation**, first introduced in the 1990s as a framework for organizations to engage in self-evaluation.[23] Donaldson[24] asserts that empowerment evaluation has transformed evaluation from an objectivist approach primarily focused on scientific rigor into a process that places stakeholder involvement and continuous learning at the forefront. The benefit of empowerment evaluation and other similar "participatory, collaborative, stakeholder-involving, and utilization-focused" approaches is that it fosters self-determination and use of the evaluation for program improvement,[23] but it has not been without controversy associated with concerns about maintaining standards of rigor and objectivity in evaluation.[25]

The second model worth noting, akin to **continuous quality improvement**, uses the Breakthrough Series Model to structure and implement multisite or multiprogram learning collaboratives in which teams focus on shared goals but conduct small tests of change (Plan, Do, Study, Act [PDSA] cycles) in their respective programs to identify changes that are promising for scale up.[26] Learning collaboratives meet periodically in learning sessions, and conduct the PDSA cycles during "action periods" between sessions. The model uses continuous data collection and assessment to determine the effects of the small changes and overall trends, and has shown tremendous success in health care and other settings.[26] Process evaluation questions include the following:

- What is working?
- What is not working?
- Do the needs of the people served match what was believed during planning?
- Is there evidence to support the assessment of needs made during the planning stage?
- Do the activities carried out by the staff match the plans for the program?
- What evidence can be found that supports the theoretical assumptions made by the program planners?[27]

Summative evaluation occurs after components of the program have been implemented and assesses the short-term and long-term intended consequences and ultimately the effects of the program on the population. According to the PRECEDE–PROCEED model,[5] **impact evaluation** examines the more immediate effects of the intervention, such as changes in participants' knowledge, attitudes, beliefs, or behaviors, and should correspond with the intervention objectives. The evaluation can also examine the extent to which the population of focus is being reached. Oftentimes, impact evaluation is a more feasible or realistic endpoint for measuring the effects of programs. **Outcome evaluation** measures the longer-term effects of the intervention and corresponds to the intervention goal. For public health programs, outcomes measured may be health status, morbidity, or mortality. It is important to note that different evaluation frameworks use these terms—outcome and impact—in reverse or interchangeably. Regardless of the evaluation framework and terms, be sure to consider both short-term and long-term effects.

Evaluation design should balance feasibility with scientific rigor. It can be challenging to identify comparison groups or obtain a large enough sample size to conduct rigorous quantitative studies. Quantitative data may include analysis of pre- and postimplementation measures and rely heavily on data quality and completeness. Quantitative methods answer questions about how much, how often, and for whom. Qualitative methods answer questions that ask how and why. Triangulation of mixed methods can increase the validity of an evaluation and help to more comprehensively understand and communicate program implementation impacts, and outcomes.

Steps in Evaluation

Evaluation starts with program design, well before the program is implemented. It is best to design an evaluation in collaboration with program designers, implementers, and recipients or participants. CDC's framework proposes the following six steps in conducting an evaluation[22]:

1. Engage stakeholders;
2. Describe the program;

3. Focus the evaluation design;
4. Gather credible evidence;
5. Justify conclusions; and
6. Ensure use and share lessons learned.

It is essential that evaluators first truly understand the program—why it was developed, the broader context, resources available, who is involved, and the expected impacts. These details are best organized in a logic model. Second, evaluators must engage and consider the needs, interests, and priorities of all stakeholders in developing evaluation questions and overall design.

These stakeholders include those involved in developing and implementing the program, individuals and communities served or affected by the program, and others who may use the results of the evaluation (funders, policymakers, designers, or implementers of other programs; see Box 7-1).

Once the evaluation is designed (step 3), methods for data collection (gathering credible evidence) should balance credibility and validity with feasibility. Gathering information about program implementation and impacts should not be burdensome for staff or program participants but needs to be sufficient to justify the conclusions (step 5). Evaluations may require both quantitative and qualitative methods and may require primary data collection (surveys, focus groups, interviews, participant observation) or examination of secondary data (program reports, abstracted client records, databases). Conclusions are the products of careful examination of the evidence (implementation and outcome data). **Program stakeholders are useful in interpreting evaluation findings and can be helpful in validating the judgments and recommendations that follow**.

Finally, the evaluation is only useful if the results are shared. As explained previously, stakeholders may provide feedback on drafts of evaluation results and can provide important contextual information without jeopardizing the validity of findings. Engaging stakeholders in finalizing evaluation results will increase the likelihood that they will be

Box 7-1. Engaging Stakeholders in Evaluation

A stakeholder is anyone who is involved in program design, operations, or implementation, or is impacted by the program (e.g., designers; implementers; current, past, or future participants; community partners; staff in other or similar programs; policymakers).

- Including stakeholders improves the validity and credibility of the evaluation. Stakeholders help to ensure that evaluation questions are relevant and on target and that methods and measures are appropriate. Stakeholders have history with the program and the broader context in which the program is embedded. Stakeholder involvement increases the sense of control over the program and the likelihood that recommendations will be implemented.
- Tips: Consider the burden on stakeholders related to their participation in the evaluation process. Ensure that stakeholders are involved in meaningful ways throughout the evaluation process. Tailor communication strategies to stakeholder groups (e.g., written, electronic, or verbal communication, in primary language and accessible language).

Source: Based on Centers for Disease Control and Prevention.[22]

used. **A plan for disseminating results is another component of the evaluation design.** Formal reports include the evaluation purpose, design, scope, and methods; description of the program and stakeholders involved; and results and recommendations. Evaluation results should be "clear, simple, action oriented, and tailored for each audience"[28] and communicated in formats that are accessible to various stakeholder groups (e.g., research briefs, reports, newsletter articles, presentations, workshops, webinars). The users of the findings can be helpful in crafting messages and helping to disseminate findings.[28]

Standards for Evaluation

High-quality evaluations are aligned with the program's underlying theory of change and also may utilize relevant theoretical models to inform methods and measures. The scope of the evaluation (e.g., community-level, program- or site-level, staff- or client-level), design (e.g., cross-sectional, case study, cohort, case–control), and methods used will be guided by evaluation questions. Evaluation in public health should also be informed by the concepts of **social ecology** and social systems, which should involve community stakeholders in a meaningful way and be shaped to fit the community.

The American Evaluation Association publishes Guiding Principles for Evaluators.[29] These standards include the following:

- **Systematic inquiry**, which ensures accuracy and credibility in methods and results, with transparency regarding the limitations of the research;
- **Competence** in designing and conducting the evaluation as well as cultural competence;
- **Integrity and honesty** in communicating with stakeholders the cost, financing, burden, limitations, changes, and in disclosing potential conflicts of interest;
- **Respect for people**, including the social and political climate, research ethics, social equity, and the potential impacts of the evaluation on stakeholders or program participants; and
- **Responsibilities for general and public welfare,** which takes into account the interests, values, and perspectives of the full range of stakeholders (with equal consideration of the needs of funders, programs, and participants/clients) in the design, conduct, and underlying assumptions of the evaluation, and in interpretation and dissemination of results.

A rigorous, high-quality evaluation also takes account of the standards put forth by CDC's Framework for Evaluation, which fall into the broad categories of **utility, feasibility, propriety,** and **accuracy**.[22] Utility standards ensure that the evaluation will be relevant and useful to program participants and stakeholders. Feasibility standards are in place to ensure that the scope and activities within an evaluation are not overreaching (i.e., "realistic, prudent, diplomatic, and frugal"[22]). The standards for propriety in evaluation address ethical considerations on behalf of those involved in the evaluation and those who could be impacted by the results. Accuracy standards have to do with the validity and adequacy of information used and conveyed by the evaluation.

PRACTICE QUESTIONS

Susie Smith is a recent graduate of the local university receiving her Master of Public Health degree with a focus in health behavior and health promotion. After graduation she secured a position as a community health educator at the local county health department. The county has a population of 20,000 individuals, most of whom are very low income with more than 50% of individuals aged 55 years and older. The majority of residents are female and white non-Hispanic. An area of need that has been identified through several needs assessments and situational analyses is residential injuries for elderly, most of which are falls. Residents are usually falling in the home (on one level) over loose rugs and things on the floor. Falls are the leading cause of emergency department visits for this age group and the leading cause of hospitalization. Susie has been tasked to develop a health promotion program for white woman, aged 55 years and older, focused on fall prevention. Behavioral objectives have been identified for this program as well. Susie is focused on using the PRECEDE–PROCEED planning model.

1. Since the health problem has been identified already, what are Susie's next steps in the planning process?
   a. Implement known interventions
   b. Determine the predisposing, enabling, and reinforcing factors after confirming objectives
   c. Determine funding for the interventions through the administrative and policy assessment
   d. Assess what policies might interfere with known interventions

Answer: b. This is the next logical step in the PRECEDE–PROCEED model once the health problem and related behaviors have been assessed. She must now establish predisposing, enabling, and reinforcing factors for the residents to help guide what needs to be included in an intervention. Choices a, c, and d come much later in the process of the model (i.e., administrative and policy assessment and intervention development).

Susie must also consider evidence-based interventions in developing her health promotion program for fall prevention among women aged 55 years and older. After considering various theory-informed interventions, she identifies that the theoretical construct of self-efficacy plays an important role in falls prevention programs as well as several constructs from Social Cognitive Theory. Working with the community coalition, she works to develop a program using Social Cognitive Theory. She uses the developed objectives to guide the development of the intervention.

2. What are the major constructs that will be important in developing the falls prevention program?

Answer: In planning the health promotion program, Susie should consider both program elements that include educational methods to impact knowledge, attitudes, beliefs, and skills and environmental change strategies to help identify ways to decrease fall risks in the community.

3. What actions should Susie take to identify existing evidence-based interventions?

Answer: Susie should start by consulting the professional literature and reviewing relevant research for existing evidence-based strategies. For example, let us say that through this she identifies several studies, but one in particular is a systematic review and meta-analysis of various controlled trials. It is revealed from these reviews that there is evidence for reduction of falls through use of risk assessments; incorporating educational interventions targeted at the individual, group, and community level; doing environmental modifications; home visits to assess fall hazards; and conducting exercise programs that focus on balance, gait, and strength. In particular, risk assessments and exercise programs appear to be most effective. Susie then identifies a draft evidence review on falls prevention interventions for the US Preventive Services Task Force after a search in the Agency for Healthcare Research and Quality Evidence-Based Practice Center Reports database. The evidence triangulates between these two comprehensive reports. Susie must assess the intervention strategies for fit within the community.

4. What core program elements should Susie select for her health promotion program intervention strategy?

Answer: Now that Susie has identified that there are several evidence-based interventions for falls prevention, she should work with her planning team to identify the relevant fit of the various core program elements: Which core elements will make a difference in behavior or outcome? Does the county have the resources (time, money, people) to implement these elements? Is this program a fit with local needs, resources, and values?

Susie decides, after much collaboration with her community coalition and review of evidence-based interventions, that the best intervention strategy includes an educational program, a home safety and falls prevention inspection with repairs and updated equipment installations, and a physician training on falls prevention education.

Susie must also consider an evaluation plan for this program. She will first want to conduct formative evaluation, ensuring that the program developed will meet the needs of the community. The formative evaluation consists of using the information gathered through the needs assessments and situational analyses that were conducted, along with information gathered from women in the community and the physicians and others who work with them, to develop the program. For example, Susie may include pilot testing materials and methods with a group of women to determine their preferred format and delivery of the program, as well as any motivators or barriers to participation. Information also needs to be collected from local physicians to inform the "physician training on patient education" component of the program. What is the current level of awareness, knowledge, and skills among physicians in addressing falls in their elderly patients? How receptive are physicians to delivering this education? What format of program delivery would be most feasible and acceptable to physicians?

5. How might formative evaluation feedback be collected from physicians?

Answer: Methods might include interviews, focus groups, surveys, observations, analysis of existing patient records, and more. The methods selected depend on the timeline, cost, stakeholder preference, and overall evaluation design. Interviews and focus groups are a great way to hear from providers about their understanding of the health issue and motivators and barriers to participating in delivering the patient education. Surveys are useful in collecting baseline data on awareness, knowledge, attitudes, and practices in order to tailor physician trainings to meet their needs. Observation of the workflow assists the program in determining the best method and approach for program delivery, and existing records may provide insight into the number of patients served, injury and health issues addressed, billing and cost, and other factors.

Susie's formative evaluation with women in the community found that, along with prevention actions they can take to create safer home environments, the housing conditions were an important determinant in falls prevention. Home repair assistance was highlighted as an overlooked need by many of the women, and thus it was added as a program component.

The evaluation plan will include process measures that will assess the extent to which the program is reaching the intended audience, that it is being implemented as planned, and that any unintended problems (or benefits!) have been identified. The process evaluation may consider quantitative measures (outputs such as the number of participants, educators, home inspections, etc.), along with qualitative input from program implementers and participants. As the program rolls out, Susie will want to review data on program activities and participation. She will also want to talk with those implementing the program as well as program participants about aspects of the program that seem to be working well versus challenges that may have arisen. The process evaluation found that participants most valued the home safety assessment and education component along with the repairs assistance. Program staff noticed that participation was highest when the home safety educator had a good rapport with the participant. An unanticipated benefit of this program component was that the home safety educator provided helpful connections to address other needs (e.g., Meals on Wheels food assistance, local community centers and senior groups, mental health and substance abuse treatment).

6. In what ways might the program be modified on the basis of this information?

Answer: The program developers may choose to build in psychosocial assessment along with a home safety checklist, additional community resources along with the injury prevention materials, and community health worker training for the home safety educators.

Susie may add an evaluation of the characteristics of the home safety educators as well as the educator–participant relationship and rapport to determine what works best. The program may also consider planning for sustainability and scale up of the program if they determine that the home educator is a valuable resource to address many concerns in this population.

Next, before fully designing and implementing the program, Susie will want to consider the desired long-term outcomes of the program, along with short- and long-term impacts. A logic model will provide a path to the North Star, or overarching outcome that the program is heading toward. The logic model also helps to lay out what measures need to be collected along the way. Determining impact and outcome measures up front provides a threefold benefit. First, it ensures that everyone involved in program planning and implementation has a clearly articulated "shared vision" of the connected inputs, activities, outputs, short-term impacts, and ultimately the long-term outcomes of the program on the populations. Second, it ensures that a data collection plan is in place before program implementation, such that pre–post measures can be collected. Third, continual data collection and examination allows the program to make changes where needed along the way. The vision for this program may ultimately be "improved health of older community residents (women aged 55 years and older)," with this program specifically focusing on a reduction in injuries from falls. Thus, Susie will want to collect a variety of data on the frequency and type of household injuries, including where and when they occur, under what circumstances, and whether there are patterns and improvements over time. Women who are not participating in the program (or are on a waitlist) may serve as a control or comparison group.

7. What short-term impact measures could be collected for women participating in this program?
   a. Rate and number of household injuries per year
   b. Knowledge, attitudes, beliefs, and skills for injury prevention
   c. Safe home environments
   d. Number of home safety inspections conducted

Answer: b and c. The short-term impacts of the program include changes in participants' knowledge, attitudes, beliefs, and skills for injury prevention. Improvements in home safety behaviors and environmental changes that have been put into place as a result of the program are also short-term measures that may be tracked through qualitative and/or quantitative measures. Choice a is a long-term impact and choice d relates to process evaluation.

CONCLUSION

Proficiency in planning and evaluation of programs in public health is critical to the success of our field. The tenants and strategies described in this chapter emphasize the important role for detailed planning and analysis, incorporating stakeholders throughout the steps. Evaluation of efforts is paramount, including the publication and presentation of not only the impact and/or outcome of the program but also how it was developed and delivered with clear explanations of the process. With this information, others can incorporate and expand upon successful public health programming and evaluation that will reach their particular populations.

REFERENCES

1. McKenzie JF, Neiger BL, Thackeray R. *Planning, Implementing, & Evaluating Health Promotion Programs: A Primer*. 6th ed. Boston, MA: Pearson; 2013.

2. McKenzie JF, Neiger BL, Thackeray R. *Planning, Implementing, & Evaluating Health Promotion Programs: A Primer*. 7th ed. Boston, MA: Pearson; 2017.

3. Center for Community Health and Development at the University of Kansas. Section 1. An overview of strategic planning or "VMOSA" (vision, mission, objectives, strategies, and action plans). Available at: http://ctb.ku.edu/en/table-of-contents/structure/strategic-planning/vmosa/main. Accessed April 26, 2018.

4. Community Preventative Services Task Force. *The Guide to Community Preventive Services*. Available at: https://www.thecommunityguide.org. Accessed April 26, 2018.

5. Green LW, Kreuter MW. *Health Program Planning: An Educational and Ecological Approach*. 4th ed. New York, NY: McGraw-Hill; 2005.

6. Bartholomew Eldredge LK, Markham CM, Ruiter RAC, Kok G, Parcel GS. *Planning Health Promotion Programs: An Intervention Mapping Approach*. 4th ed. San Francisco, CA: Jossey-Bass; 2016.

7. Intervention Mapping Summer Course. Intervention mapping. Available at: https://interventionmapping.com. Accessed April 27, 2018.

8. Agency for Healthcare Research and Quality. EPC evidence-based reports. Available at: https://www.ahrq.gov/research/findings/evidence-based-reports/index.html. Accessed April 27, 2018.

9. McMaster University, National Collaborating Centre for Methods and Tools. Health evidence. Available at: https://www.healthevidence.org. Accessed April 27, 2018.

10. Cochrane Library. Available at: http://www.cochranelibrary.com. Accessed April 27, 2018.

11. National Cancer Institute. Research-tested intervention programs (RTIPs). Available at: https://rtips.cancer.gov/rtips/index.do. Accessed March 19, 2018.

12. Centers for Disease Control and Prevention. Effective interventions: HIV prevention that works. Available at: https://effectiveinterventions.cdc.gov. Accessed April 27, 2018.

13. Substance Abuse and Mental Health Services Administration. National Registry of Evidence-Based Programs and Practices. Available at: http://www.samhsa.gov/nrepp. Accessed September 4, 2018.

14. Bensley RJ, Brookins-Fisher J, eds. *Community Health Education Methods: A Practical Guide.* 3rd ed. Sudbury, MA: Jones & Bartlett Publishers; 2009.

15. Center for Community Health and Development at the University of Kansas. Community Tool Box. Available at: http://ctb.ku.edu/en/dothework/tools_tk_1.aspx. Accessed April 15, 2018.

16. Kok G, Gottlieb NH, Peters GJ, et al. A taxonomy of behavior change methods: an intervention mapping approach. *Health Psychol Rev.* 2016;10(3):297–312.

17. Peters G-J. A taxonomy of behavior change methods: an intervention mapping approach. Supplemental materials. 2015. Available at: https://osf.io/sqtuz. Accessed September 4, 2018.

18. Effectivebehaviorchange.com. Behavior change made accessible. Available at: https://effectivebehaviorchange.com. Accessed April 27, 2018.

19. Issel LM, Wells R. *Health Program Planning and Evaluation: A Practical, Systematic Approach for Community Health.* 4th ed. Burlington, MA: Jones & Bartlett Learning; 2018.

20. Center for Community Health and Development at the University of Kansas. Chapter 18. Deciding where to start. Community Tool Box. Available at: https://ctb.ku.edu/en/table-of-contents/analyze/where-to-start. Accessed April 27, 2018.

21. Patton MQ. *Utilization-Focused Evaluation.* 4th ed. Thousand Oaks, CA: Sage Publications; 2008.

22. Centers for Disease Control and Prevention. A framework for program evaluation. Available at: https://www.cdc.gov/eval/framework/index.htm. Accessed April 27, 2018.

23. Patton MQ. Toward distinguishing empowerment evaluation and placing it in a larger context. *Eval Pract.* 1997;18(2):147–163.

24. Donaldson SI. Empowerment evaluation: an approach that has literally altered the landscape of evaluation. *Eval Program Plann.* 2017;63(1):136–137.

25. Stufflebeam DL. Empowerment evaluation, objectivist evaluation, and evaluation standards: where the future of evaluation should not go and where it needs to go. *Eval Pract.* 1994;15(3): 321–338.

26. Institute for Healthcare Improvement. The Breakthrough Series: IHI's Collaborative Model for Achieving Breakthrough Improvement. 2003. Available at: http://www.IHI.org. Accessed June 18, 2018.

27. Posavac EJ. *Program Evaluation: Methods and Case Studies.* 8th ed. New York, NY: Routledge; 2016.

28. Gagnon ML. Moving knowledge to action through dissemination and exchange. *J Clin Epidemiol.* 2011;64(1):25–31.

29. American Evaluation Association. American Evaluation Association guiding principles for evaluators. Available at: http://www.eval.org/p/cm/ld/fid=51. Accessed April 29, 2018.

8

Program Management

Sandra Potthoff, PhD

INTRODUCTION

"Leadership" (Chapter 3) describes the difference between **leadership** and **management**. Leadership is "doing the right thing," whereas management is "doing things right."[1] Key leadership responsibilities entail articulating a bold vision; being externally focused on the changing landscape to position the organization on a strategic direction to succeed in its mission, vision, and values; and engaging and inspiring key internal and external stakeholders to help achieve the organization's mission, goals, and objectives.[2-4]

The "doing things right" of management focuses on aligning and integrating internal organizational operations to the organization's strategy, strategic plan, goals, and objectives in order to drive performance excellence.[2-4] The Baldrige Performance Excellence Framework provides system-based self-assessment criteria that support an organization's ability to improve in aligning and integrating strategy and operations.[5]

Aligning and integrating organizational strategic and operational goals, objectives, and processes requires strong program management skills, particularly those related to budgeting and financial management, securing resources, and program implementation and evaluation. This chapter focuses on the following Association of Schools and Programs of Public Health Program Management tasks critical for organizational effectiveness:

- Budgeting and financial management
  - ❑ Task 1: Develop program or organizational budgets with justification.
  - ❑ Task 2: Defend a programmatic or organizational budget.
  - ❑ Task 3: Operate programs within current and forecasted budget constraints.
  - ❑ Task 4: Respond to changes in financial resources.
- Securing resources to support programmatic activities
  - ❑ Task 5: Develop proposals to secure financial support.
  - ❑ Task 6: Participate in the development of contracts or other agreements for the provision of services.
  - ❑ Task 7: Ensure implementation of contracts or other agreements for the provision of services.
  - ❑ Task 8: Leverage existing resources for program management.
  - ❑ Task 9: Identify methods for assuring health program sustainability.

- Implementing, evaluating, and improving programs to improve the public's health
  - ❑ Task 10: Give constructive feedback to others about their performance on the team.
  - ❑ Task 11: Develop monitoring and evaluation frameworks to assess programs.
  - ❑ Task 12: Implement a community health plan.
  - ❑ Task 13: Implement programs to ensure community health.

Begun and Malcolm describe such tasks as those related to driving for execution and continuous improvement in public health,[4] while Honoré and Costich include them as public health financial competencies.[6]

MAJOR CONTENT

Budgeting and Financial Management

A vision without resources is a hallucination.[7]

Organizations typically develop an operational plan for a given time horizon (e.g., three years) that flows from their strategic plan, goals, and objectives. They also engage in an annual planning process that focuses on the organization's upcoming **fiscal year**. A fiscal year is the annual timeframe used for financial accounting purposes (e.g., July 1 through June 30, or January 1 through December 31). Operational plans cascade down into sub-plans for departments within an organization. Similarly, specific programs carried out by an organization will have their associated operational plans.

Operational plans require **budgets**, which are detailed financial plans comprising estimates of **revenues** or **income**, money generated by the activities of the operational plan or received from such sources as grants, and **expenses** or **costs**, money being expended on resources required to carry out the operational plan. The process of estimating the coming year's revenues and costs is called **budgeting**. The budgeting process occurs annually to prepare for the upcoming fiscal year of the organization. Budgeting is the financial part of the planning process that ensures short-term financial obligations of the organization are met, and long-term sustainability of an organization is secured.

The Public Health Finance and Management Web site provides a series of tutorials related to public health budgeting and financial management.[8-13]

Task 1: Develop Program or Organizational Budgets With Justification

Public health managers should be competent in developing organizational and program budgets. Budgets require detailed information on all revenues and expenses by category. Each category usually has its own separate line in the budget, which is referred to as a **line item**.[10]

Examples of **revenue categories** include money generated by charging fees to provide services, grant and contract funding, sales, investment income, and donations. Examples of **expense categories** include staffing costs and fringe benefit costs (e.g., vacation, paid time off, health insurance), supply and equipment costs, rent, utilities, printing, postage, and travel costs. Staffing costs are typically estimated on a **full-time-equivalent (FTE)** basis. FTE staffing calculations typically assume a 40-hour work week, or 2,080 hours per year (52 weeks per year times 40 hours per week).[10]

An organization's total revenues should exceed or meet total expenses. If they do not, then the organization has a **budget deficit**, and it is experiencing what is called a "loss." This is not good. In for-profit organizations, the excess of revenues over expenses is called "profit." In not-for-profit organizations, it is called **margin**.[10] Hence, there is the saying "no margin, no mission."

Public health organizations are typically not-for-profit. Therefore, profit maximization would not be a goal of the organization; having a positive margin or at least a balanced budget should be. A balanced budget means that the organization's total revenues are equal to its total expenses, so its margin would be equal to (or very close to) zero. The formula to calculate the margin is margin = total revenues – total expenses.

Agencies that provide funding opportunities through grants or contracts will have a **budget template** provided in their funding application materials that must be followed when submitting an application. Example budget templates can be found on the Internet by using the search term "organizational budget template." Details of each revenue source (if applicable) and each required program resource that generates expenses in support of your proposed program must be described. In addition, a **budget justification** must be provided that explains why each resource is needed and provides the assumptions and calculations that were used to generate dollar amounts for each line item of the budget. A sample budget justification format for the Centers for Disease Control and Prevention can be found at https://www.cdc.gov/healthyyouth/fundedpartners/pdf/budget_guidelines.pdf.[14]

Task 2: Defend a Programmatic or Organizational Budget

Public health professionals are fiduciary stewards of the public's funds entrusted to their organizations to improve the public's health. Thus, public health budgets are subject to scrutiny by organizational leaders, funding agencies, legislators, and the public. For a budget to be defensible, it must be transparent, logical, and justifiable. As a starting point, it should be clear how the budget ties to the organization's strategy and operational plan. If a new project or program is being proposed, it should have a **business plan** that provides financial, operational, and marketing detail so that its costs and benefits can be assessed.[11]

If budget cuts are being proposed or if a particular initiative risks not getting funded, you need to be very clear about the implications of the funding failure for what the organization will not be able to accomplish. You will need to explain the program cuts that will be required, what staff and other stakeholders will be affected, the impact on public health outcomes, and the line items in the budget that will be affected.

Proactive approaches to defending budgets include documenting the "value proposition" of programs and activities. Given limited money, time, people, or other resources, which programs should receive funding? Methods to answer this question include **benchmarking,** calculating **return on investment (ROI)**, and **economic evaluation**.

Benchmarking is a performance measurement process in which you find organizations that provide programs and services similar to yours and that are considered "best in class" in their processes and outcomes in delivering them. You then compare your organization's financial performance, processes, and outcomes against those of these external organizations. This enables your organization to both continuously improve by learning from top performers, and to justify how your organization compares with those who are considered "best in class."[15,16]

ROI is a financial ratio that is used to measure program efficiency. ROI compares the costs of a program with the financial savings generated by that program, calculated as

$$\frac{\text{Financial Savings From Program} - \text{Cost of Program}}{\text{Cost of Program}} \times 100\%$$

The higher the ROI, the more financial benefit is accruing from the invested monies. An ROI of less than or equal to 0% means that there is no financial gain from the investment in the program. In public health and health care, savings can sometimes accrue to an entity different from the one funding the program. Also, outcomes achieved through public health investments cannot always be quantifiable as financial.[11,17]

Economic evaluation considers both costs and outcomes of a program, with costs in the numerator and outcomes in the denominator. But how should outcomes be measured? There is a variety of economic evaluation ratios, each of which measures outcomes differently. **Cost–benefit analysis** quantifies tangible and "soft" outcomes into a monetary number. **Cost-effectiveness analysis** measures program outcomes in similar units across programs (e.g., life-years saved) rather than trying to quantify the outcome in dollars. **Cost-utility analysis** measures outcomes by using a standardized morbidity or mortality measure, often a metric called a quality-adjusted life-year.[18,19]

Task 3: Operate Programs Within Current and Forecasted Budget Constraints

Budgets are not tools for accountants. They are tools for managers to ensure that they are using resources wisely and efficiently. Budgets are estimates or projections of revenues and expenses. Thus, they must be monitored on a regular basis (e.g., monthly) to compare planned revenues and expenses with actual revenues generated and expenses incurred. If actual performance is greatly different from planned, managers must investigate reasons for the discrepancy and take corrective action.

Variance reports are monthly budget reports that compare the *budgeted* revenues and expenses with the *actual* revenues and expenses for each line item in the budget.[10] The timeframes typically reported in a variance report are the budgeted and actual comparisons for month-to-date and year-to-date for the current year and the previous fiscal year. Variance reports will often also include a column that calculates the percent variance to help the manager quickly assess whether the variance is positive, called a favorable variance (actual is better than budgeted), or negative, called an unfavorable variance (actual is worse than budgeted):

Revenue % Variance = (Actual Revenues − Budget Revenues) / Budget Revenues
Cost % Variance = (Budgeted Costs − Actual Costs) / Budgeted Costs

The layout of a typical variance report will have the columns of data found in Table 8-1. The manager needs to review the monthly variance reports to determine if corrective action is needed and, if so, where. The manager must look at the variance in each of the revenue and expense line items to identify where in the budget the unfavorable variances lie. Are actual salary expenses exceeding budgeted expenses? Is there a problem in supply expenses? If some revenue is generated by fees that are generated by visits, is the volume of visits less than expected, resulting in less fee revenue? Did some projected grant funding not come in because the organization was not successful in securing the funding? Similarly, if favorable variances are occurring, can the organization study the underlying reasons to identify possible ways to sustain this improved performance?

Variance reports must also be reviewed for specific program or project budgets. These variance reports must be tracked to ensure that funds are being expended as expected by category and that project fund balances are sufficient to carry out the promised scope of work for the grant period of funding.

Table 8-1. Columns of Data

Month-to-Date (MTD)					Year-to-Date (YTD)				
Actual MTD Oct. 2017	Budget MTD Oct. 2017	Variance F (U)	Variance % F (U)	Actual MTD Oct. 2016	Actual YTD Oct. 2017	Budget YTD Oct. 2017	Variance F (U)	Variance % F (U)	Actual YTD Oct. 2016

Note: F = favorable; U = unfavorable.

In public health organizations, it is critical that **restricted revenues** obtained via grants or contracts to carry out a specified scope of work be used just for those purposes. Restricted funds cannot be used to cover shortfalls in revenue streams or cost overruns for other programs. Very careful records must be maintained to ensure that internal and external audits of the funds can prove they were used only as intended.[20]

Task 4: Respond to Changes in Financial Resources

If financial resources become constrained, managers have two levers—grow revenues or reduce costs. Reducing costs requires understanding the organization's cost structure. There are two ways to define costs:

1. **Direct** versus **indirect or overhead costs**
2. **Variable** versus **fixed** costs

These two different ways of classifying costs are important in calculating two financial metrics that provide insights into financial sustainability of a program. These financial metrics are the **contribution margin** and the **breakeven point**.[9]

Direct Versus Overhead Costs

Costs that would not be incurred any longer if a program were to disappear because the resources generating those costs would no longer be needed are called **direct costs**. Examples of direct costs are a program's staffing costs (assuming the staff would be laid off if the program were discontinued).

Other resources are needed to support the entire portfolio of services provided by an organization. Examples include the salaries and benefits of the leadership team; the accounting, finance, human resources, housekeeping, and information technology staff; office computer costs; and building costs (e.g., rent, heat, light, phone, Internet). The costs of these shared resources must be accounted for when one is creating budgets by allocating them to the various services provided by the organization or to the departments of the organization. These costs are called **indirect or overhead costs**. These costs are incurred regardless of whether an individual program is discontinued. There is a variety of approaches that can be used to allocate overhead costs to the programs being delivered.[21] For federal grants, the overhead component of the budget is typically called facilities and administration.

Variable Versus Fixed Costs

Variable costs are incurred only when resources are used to provide the services of the program. If the volume of services provided decreases, then the variable cost to provide the service decreases. Program supplies, for example, are generally a variable cost. **Fixed costs** are costs that are incurred regardless of the volume of services provided. Even if the

Table 8-2. Examples of Types of Costs

	Direct	Overhead
Variable	Supplies used for each unit of service provided, staff costs if paid per unit of service provided	Electricity costs that vary on the basis of units of service provided
Fixed	Staff costs if paid an annual salary regardless of volume of units of service provided	Rent, insurance, management support services

program provided half of the volume of services that was projected, it would still incur all of the fixed costs.

Overhead costs are most often fixed costs, but direct costs could be either fixed or variable costs. If staff hired to deliver a particular program are paid a set salary regardless of the volume of services they provide, then these staffing costs are fixed, direct costs. If staff are paid on a per-unit-of-service-provided basis, then staffing costs will vary depending on the volume of services delivered, and they are a variable, direct cost. See Table 8-2 for examples of types of costs.

When providing services, it is important to compare the revenue generated per unit of service with the variable cost per unit of service. This is called the **contribution margin**, and is calculated as

Contribution Margin = Revenue per Unit of Service − Variable Cost per Unit of Service

If the contribution margin is negative (unit variable cost exceeds unit revenue), you are losing money on each unit of service provided, and no amount of program growth will enable the program to break even (defined in the next paragraph). This is not good! You cannot lose money on every unit of service you provide and "stay in business." To have a positive contribution margin, either revenue per unit of service must increase or variable costs per unit of service must decrease.

If the contribution margin is positive (unit revenue exceeds unit variable cost), then the program is "making money" on each unit of service provided. This means that your total revenue is exceeding your total variable cost. This is good! But, is the program generating enough revenue to also cover its fixed costs? This is called the **breakeven point**, and is calculated as

Breakeven Point: Total Revenue = Total Variable Costs + Total Fixed Costs

If the program's total revenue is less than the sum of the program's total variable and fixed costs, the program is not breaking even (i.e., it is losing money). Algebra can be used to calculate how many units of service must be provided to cover a program's fixed costs in order to break even.

These two financial metrics—contribution margin and breakeven point—will help managers identify how much additional revenue must be generated or how much fixed or variable costs will need to be decreased, if financial viability is to be maintained.

Securing Resources to Support Programmatic Activities

Financial sustainability requires revenue streams to support the work of an organization's mission. Revenues for public health organizations can come from a variety of sources, including government appropriations, federal and state contracts and grants, foundation grants, direct provision of services for which payments are received, and philanthropic donations from private companies or individuals. Thus, a portfolio of revenue streams must be managed for public health organizations to be successful.

Federal dollars that support public health services and programs flow through federal agencies to state, county, local, and other public health organizations. This funding can be one of several different types. **Block grants** are relatively large sums of money that the federal government passes through to states, with broad discretion on how the states can spend the funds. **Categorical funds**, on the other hand, are restricted to being spent on specific programs or initiatives. Some categorical funds are distributed as grants based on pass-through formulas (e.g., infant mortality rates), while other categorical funds will be competitively awarded for specific projects through a grant application process.[8]

Funds from state, county, or local governments can include those allocated through an appropriations process, through formulas to fund public health agencies for specific services, or through a taxing mechanism (e.g., local property tax line item) that allocates funds to local public health agencies. Community foundations and organizations also fund public health activities either through direct donations or through a competitive grant application process.[8]

For public health organizations that provide health care services, funds can be generated through billing recipients of the services or their health care insurance provider. Reimbursement methods can either be capitated or fee-for-service. **Capitation** means the service provider receives a set amount of revenue per person enrolled per time period (typically per member per month, known as PMPM), regardless of the volume of services delivered to each person. **Fee-for-service** reimbursement can be either retrospective or prospective. In a retrospective method, the service provider is reimbursed on the basis of their prices charged (or a negotiated discount rate to the charges). For prospective payment, the service provider may be paid a set amount on the basis of the diagnosis of the patient, regardless of the cost of services provided, on a per-day (per-diem) basis, or on a per-procedure basis.[8]

Public health leaders need to understand the mix of revenue streams that support their organization's work and the sustainability of their mix of funding sources. Funders can change their priorities, which can result in budget cuts or loss of funding for core programs. When revenue shortfalls occur, managers must make hard decisions that are consistent with the organization's mission.

Task 5: Develop Proposals to Secure Financial Support

Organizations that sustain themselves for the long term excel at the intersection of knowing what they are passionate about (mission-driven), what they can be the best at, and the financial or "business" model that will sustain their work.[2-4] A key to success in seeking funding is to understand the work and activities that are central to an organization's core mission and to seek funding for that work. If a funding agency is soliciting proposals in an area that is not a part of an organization's core mission and competencies, it is not in the best interest of the organization's long-term viability to chase that funding opportunity. If it does, it risks losing its ability to focus on and execute what it does well. Sometimes part of the scope of work requested in a grant opportunity is an organization's core competency while the remainder is not. In these situations, it is important to develop partnerships and collaborations with other community organizations (see "Collaboration and Partnership" [Chapter 6]) to seek funding jointly.

There are a number of online resources that describe how to write proposals to federal and state agencies or private foundations to seek funding support.[22,23] Each funding agency or foundation has its own requirements for the outline of the grant proposal and requirements for submission. A typical format will include an introduction, a statement of the problem that your project addresses, a narrative description of your proposed project, the goals of the project, the measurable objectives and outcomes of the project, the evaluation plan, the timeline of tasks and deliverables, and the budget and budget justification for the project. Federal government agencies require a number of registration steps to submit proposals.[24]

Federal government funding opportunities are posted on the Web site https://grants. gov.[25] State agencies with funding opportunities can be found on their respective Web sites. A comprehensive database of private foundations is available online for a subscription fee; public and university libraries may have a subscription so that organizations can access it for free.[26] When researching potential funders, it is important to talk to them to describe your initiative or project. This will ensure that you are identifying the potential funder whose targeted funding priority areas are the best fit.

Task 6: Participate in the Development of Contracts or Other Agreements for the Provision of Services

Funding opportunities to which organizations can apply may be either **contracts** or **grants**. **Contracts** are legally binding agreements used by government agencies to procure services in support of activities the government wishes to carry out.[21,27-29] The agency describes the required scope of work, the timeline in which the work must be completed, and the required deliverables (products) throughout and upon completion of the contract. The agency solicits bids from organizations to complete that scope of work and abide by the requirements. By contrast, the proposed idea and scope of work for **grants** are developed by the organization seeking grant funding. Government agencies, private foundations, and businesses and corporations utilize grants submitted by organizations as a mechanism to fund projects of interest.

Task 7: Ensure Implementation of Contracts or Other Agreements for the Provision of Services

If an organization is awarded a contract, it is legally obligated to conduct the scope of work as promised for the agreed-upon contracted financial amount and must file frequent reports as specified in the contract regarding completion of promised scope of work. If the organization does not fulfill the scope of work as delineated in the contract, it may be subject to legal action or financial penalties. One federal agency often involved in soliciting contracts for work related to public health is the US Department of Health and Human Services, which includes the Centers for Disease Control and Prevention.[21,29] Their Web sites describe the contracting process and they post contract opportunities to which organizations can apply. Other examples include the US Department of Health and Human Services Health Resources and Services Administration and the Maternal and Child Health Block Grants, which require recipients to track and report on specified outcome and performance measures.[30]

Task 8: Leverage Existing Resources for Program Management

Public health organizations typically have myriad programs they offer concurrently to a variety of different stakeholders, clients, and the public. In addition, there may be other organizations that provide similar or complementary services in the community. It is important that organizations look both internally and externally in ensuring they are leveraging existing resources to carry out their work. Internally, organizations need to keep their overhead and fixed costs as low as possible in administering their portfolio of programs. Externally, organizations need to partner with other community organizations who are doing similar work to fully leverage the potential scope and reach of their programs. "Collaboration and Partnership" (Chapter 6) describes partnerships in more detail.

Task 9: Identify Methods for Assuring Health Program Sustainability

Health programs require resources, and there are numerous programs competing for those resources. Sustaining a health program requires a variety of methods to ensure **sustainability**. First, a necessary, but not sufficient condition for sustainability is that the program is evidence-based and effective as demonstrated by both formative and summative evaluation with identified goals, objectives, and metrics. Second, quality-management principles (see Task 11) must be in place to ensure that the programs are continuously monitored and improved upon, both in terms of process (e.g., who is served and how are they served) and outcomes (measurable impacts of the program). But sustainability requires more than this. Studies have documented that there is a variety of factors that may affect program sustainability, including program evaluation and adaption, public health impacts, strategic planning, political support, funding stability, communications, partnerships, and organizational capacity.[31-33] Sustainability assessment tools are available to help guide managers in sustaining their health programs.[34,35] It is important to address issues of sustainability at the outset of any new program, as many funding agencies require a sustainability plan in their grant proposal applications.

Implementing, Evaluating, and Improving Programs to Improve the Public's Health

Implementing, evaluating, and improving programs to improve the public's health requires successful execution and continuous improvement. In addition, much of the work in improving the public's health is accomplished through collaborative teams. Hence, effective team management and teamwork are crucial to successful program implementation, evaluation, and improvement. Two other chapters in this review guide cover these topics in detail. "Program Planning and Evaluation" (Chapter 7) provides in-depth detail on implementing, evaluating, and improving programs. "Collaboration and Partnership" (Chapter 6) describes how to successfully engage stakeholders, community partners, and others in collaborative efforts and partnerships. Thus, the remaining four tasks described next have extensive coverage in the other chapters. The additional information will therefore focus on methods for team performance and continuous improvement.

Task 10: Give Constructive Feedback to Others About Their Performance on the Team

High-functioning teams do not happen by accident. Teams go through stages of development as members are brought together to achieve a goal. As described by Tuckman, these **team stages** include forming, storming, norming, and performing.[36] Relationships must form among team members; conflict and cliques may occur as the team begins to focus on its tasks and goals; and team leaders must work on helping the team develop trust, support, and group identity; and once that occurs, the team can achieve peak performance. Allowing time for the forming stage for team members working on public health issues is particularly important as team members are diverse in terms of professional background, sector of the community, race, and social class.

Effective teams also require effective **team management techniques**. These techniques include methods for running productive meetings, generating effective discussions and decisions, creating effective recordkeeping, using team roles (e.g., project leader, meeting leader, timekeeper, recorder) and executing through effective planning.[37-39]

Effective team performance also requires holding yourself and other team members accountable.[40] This requires ongoing evaluation of both team performance and individual team member performance. Both qualitative and quantitative methods can be utilized.[41] The team leader needs to continuously observe both whole-team dynamics and individual team member behavior or performance issues and know how to conduct productive team or individual private conversations when issues arise that need to be addressed.[40,42] The purpose of these discussions is to give feedback that helps the team and team members grow professionally and personally.

Task 11: Develop Monitoring and Evaluation Frameworks to Assess Programs

Public health agencies are increasingly using **quality improvement** (**QI**) tools and techniques to systematically study and improve their programs, activities, and efforts.[39,43,44] QI uses continuous, repeatable, defined processes and measurement methods. A common QI framework used in industry and increasingly in public health is the **plan-do-study-act** (**PDSA**) process (sometimes called plan-do-check-act).[44,45] The "study" phase of the process focuses on measuring program impacts, trends, benefits, and unintended consequences. PDSA is a continuous change management process that complements the steps of the logic model and PRECEDE–PROCEED (predisposing, reinforcing, and enabling constructs in educational/ecological diagnosis and evaluation [PRECEDE]–policy, regulatory, and organizational constructs in educational and environmental development [PROCEED]) model described in "Program Planning and Evaluation" (Chapter 7). As shown in the Baldrige Performance Excellence framework referenced at the beginning of this chapter,[5] monitoring and evaluation also require a data management system with clearly defined process and outcome measures, with accompanying processes for data collection and knowledge management.

Tasks 12 and 13: Implement a Community Health Plan and Implement Programs to Ensure Community Health

As described in "Collaboration and Partnership" (Chapter 6), plans and programs to improve the health of communities are increasingly relying on collaboration across community partners spanning diverse sectors such as education, health, public health, city planning, and economic development. As such, implementation competencies span traditional **project management** skills as well as **backbone organization** roles. Project management competencies include both people skills and technical skills. People skills are needed to build trust and promote communication across stakeholders. Technical skills include seeing the big picture down to developing detailed implementation action plans that describe the scope of work to be completed, deliverables, tasks, assignments, timelines, and due dates.[46] **Flow charts** and **Gantt charts** are examples of QI tools that are frequently used in developing implementation plans. Flow charts document visually the sequential order in which activities are carried out.[37–39,47] Gantt charts use horizontal bar charts to visually represent the list of activities that must be completed, with the timeline of when they will be completed.[47] There is a professional organization called the Project Management Institute that supports certification in project management.[48]

Successful development and implementation of cross-sector community plans and programs are often supported by a backbone organization that provides the infrastructure and know-how to convene and coordinate the ongoing collaboration and evolving initiatives. There are six functions of a backbone organization:

1. Guide vision and strategy.
2. Support aligned activities.
3. Establish shared measurement practices.
4. Build public will.
5. Advance policy.
6. Mobilize funding.[49,50]

PRACTICE QUESTIONS

You are the administrator of a community clinic in a rural county with limited access to preventive services. The county public health department has received a grant to purchase a mobile digital mammography screening van. The regional health care system has agreed to provide as community benefit the cost of the radiologist's time to interpret the digital mammograms, with the digital images being sent nightly to their facility to be read. The county has asked that your clinic be responsible for the daily operations and expenses of providing the digital mammography screening services. They have asked you to put together a document that shows the daily work flow and tasks for the screening service, a staffing plan, and a budget showing assumptions of projected revenues and expenses.

1. The clinic is responsible for paying for the van insurance and the service maintenance contract for the digital mammography equipment. These costs do not fluctuate on the basis of the number of digital mammograms performed. What type of costs are these?
   a. Fixed costs
   b. Variable costs

Answer: a. Costs that do not vary on the basis of the number of units produced are considered fixed costs.

2. There are two digital scanning machines on the van, each of which requires a technologist to operate. Each day will require 20 hours of technologist time (8 hours per technologist per machine, plus 1 hour each at the start of the day to set up and 1 hour each at the end of the day to close down). The mobile van will be operating 6 days per week, 52 weeks per year. Assuming a 40-hour work week is full-time, how many technologist FTEs are required for this workload?

    a. 2 FTEs

    b. 3 FTEs

    c. 4 FTEs

Answer: b. Each day requires 20 hours times 6 days per week is 120 hours of technology time per week times 52 weeks per year = 6,240 hours. 1 FTE is 52 weeks per year times 40 hours per week = 2,080 hours. 6,240/2,080 = 3 FTEs.

3. If the technologists are not paid a salary, but instead are paid according to the number of mammograms they complete, what type of cost would this be?

    a. Variable direct cost

    b. Fixed direct cost

    c. Variable overhead cost

    d. Fixed overhead cost

Answer: a. It is a variable direct cost. The technologists are involved in providing direct service, so they are a direct cost. If they are paid on the basis of production rather than a fixed salary, then their costs are variable on the basis of production.

4. You estimate that the revenue the clinic will receive per mammogram is $100. The variable cost per mammogram is $70. You estimate that you will pay a $60,000-per-year fixed salary to each of your three FTE technologists ($180,000 total) and an additional $120,000 in fixed costs for insurance, equipment service contracts, etc.

a. What is the contribution margin per mammogram?

Answer: Contribution margin = revenue per unit of service – variable cost per unit of service = $100 – $70 = $30.

b. How many mammograms will need to be done annually to break even?

Answer: The breakeven point is where total revenue = total variable costs + total fixed costs.

- Total revenue = revenue per mammogram × number of mammograms.
- Total variable costs = variable cost per mammogram × number of mammograms.
- Total fixed costs = 3 staff × $60,000 per year + $120,000 = $300,000.

Using algebra, the breakeven point = (revenue per mammogram – variable cost per mammogram) × number of mammograms = total fixed costs.

Number of mammograms = total fixed costs/(revenue per mammogram − variable cost per mammogram) = $300,000/($100 − $70) = 10,000 mammograms annually is the breakeven point.

5. Assuming each digital scan takes 30 minutes and that there are two staffed mammography machines for 8 hours a day, 6 days a week, 52 weeks a year, is it possible to attain the breakeven point?

Answer: Almost, but no. Assuming 8 hours per day × 2 scans per hour × 2 machines = 32 mammograms per day × 6 days per week × 52 weeks per year = 9,984 mammograms per year of capacity. Breakeven is 10,000 mammograms. Even if the van runs at 100% of capacity, which is not realistic, the capacity limit is 9,984 mammograms.

6. Why would you review monthly variance reports produced about the van's ongoing operations?
   a. To determine who to blame for costs that are too high
   b. To compare actual revenues and costs with what was planned in the budget
   c. To calculate the contribution margin of the program
   d. To develop a budget justification

Answer: b. Monthly budget variance reports help managers identify where actual revenues and expenses are not occurring as planned in the original budget. This enables managers to identify areas (e.g., staffing, supplies, revenue generation) that may need attention because there is an unfavorable variance that is identified in the variance report.

7. Which tool would be the most appropriate to use to visually show the activities that need to be conducted each day by the technologists to carry out their work?
   a. Logic model
   b. PRECEDE–PROCEED planning model
   c. Flow chart
   d. PDSA cycle

Answer: c. Flow charts are QI tools that document the steps of a process visually so that they can be implemented in a systematic, repeatable manner.

CONCLUSION

This chapter provides a summary and references for the 13 ASPPH program management tasks. These tasks span (1) budgeting and financial management, (2) securing resources to support programmatic activities, and (3) implementing, evaluating, and improving programs to improve the public's health. They provide public health professionals with the technical and QI skills necessary to succeed in an era of increased accountability for the wise use of public resources.

REFERENCES

1. Warren B, Nanus B. *Leaders: The Strategies for Taking Charge.* New York, NY: Harper and Row; 1985:21.

2. Collins J. *Good to Great: Why Some Companies Make the Leap . . . and Others Don't.* New York, NY: HarperBusiness; 2001.

3. Collins J. *Good to Great and the Social Sectors: A Monograph to Accompany Good to Great.* New York, NY: HarperBusinsess; 2006.

4. Begun JW, Malcolm JK. *Leading Public Health: A Competency Framework.* New York, NY: Springer Publishing Company; 2014.

5. National Institute of Standards and Technology, Baldrige Performance Excellence Program. How Baldrige works. Available at: https://www.nist.gov/baldrige/how-baldrige-works. Accessed August 4, 2017.

6. Honoré PA, Costich FJ. Public health financial management competencies. *J Public Health Manag Pract.* 2009;14(4):311–318.

7. Friedman TL. Live bad, go green. *New York Times.* July 8, 2007. Available at: http://www.nytimes.com/2007/07/08/opinion/08friedman.html?mcubz=3. Accessed August 4, 2017.

8. Public Health Finance and Management. Public health finance tutorial series module I: financing public health services. Available at: http://www.publichealthfinance.org/media/file/PHFM_Finance_Tutorial_I.pdf. Accessed August 4, 2017.

9. Public Health Finance and Management. Public health finance tutorial series module II: estimating costs and margins. Available at: http://www.publichealthfinance.org/media/file/PHFM_Finance_Tutorial_II.pdf. Accessed August 4, 2017.

10. Public Health Finance and Management. Public health finance tutorial series module III: financial planning and budgeting. Available at: http://www.publichealthfinance.org/media/file/PHFM_Finance_Tutorial_III.pdf. Accessed August 4, 2017.

11. Public Health Finance and Management. Public health finance tutorial series module IV: financial evaluation of new program initiatives. Available at: http://www.publichealthfinance.org/media/file/PHFM_Finance_Tutorial_IV.pdf. Accessed August 4, 2017.

12. Public Health Finance and Management. Public health finance tutorial series module V: financial reporting. Available at: http://www.publichealthfinance.org/media/file/PHFM_Finance_Tutorial_V.pdf. Accessed August 4, 2017.

13. Public Health Finance and Management. Public health finance tutorial series module VI: assessing financial performance. Available at: http://www.publichealthfinance.org/media/file/PHFM_Finance_Tutorial_VI.pdf. Accessed August 4, 2017.

14. Centers for Disease Control and Prevention. Guidelines for budget preparation. Available at: https://www.cdc.gov/healthyyouth/fundedpartners/pdf/budget_guidelines.pdf. Accessed December 2, 2017.

15. Ettorchi-Tardy A, Levif M, Michel P. Benchmarking: a method for continuous quality improvement in health. *Healthc Policy.* 2012;7(4):e101–e119.

16. Ontario Health Promotion Email Bulletin. Benchmarking as a tool for public health and health promotion. Available at: http://www.ohpe.ca/node/149. Accessed December 1, 2017.

17. Teutsch SM, Koo D, Grosse SD. Return on investment and economic evaluation. In: Michener JL, Koo D, Castrucci BC, Sprague JB, eds. *The Practical Playbook.* New York, NY: Oxford Press; 2016:225–232.

18. Rabarison KM, Bish CL, Massoudi MS, Giles WH. Economic evaluation enhances public health decision making. *Front Public Health.* 2015;3:164.

19. Weinstein MC, Torrance G, McGuire A. QALYs: the basics. *Value Health.* 2009;12(suppl 1): S5–S9.

20. Johnson S. Tracking and managing restricted funds. Social Solutions. Available at: http://www.socialsolutions.com/blog/tracking-and-managing-restricted-funds. Accessed May 3, 2018.

21. US Department of Health and Human Services. Grants and contracts. Available at: https://www.hhs.gov/grants/index.html. Accessed August 28, 2017.

22. University of Kansas Center for Community Health and Development. Chapter 42 Section 4. Applying for a grant: the general approach. Community Tool Box. Available at: http://ctb.ku.edu/en/table-of-contents/finances/grants-and-financial-resources/grant-application/main. Accessed August 30, 2017.

23. University of Kansas Center for Community Health and Development. Chapter 42 Section 5. Writing a grant. Community Tool Box. Available at: http://ctb.ku.edu/en/table-of-contents/finances/grants-and-financial-resources/writing-a-grant/main. Accessed August 30, 2017.

24. US Department of Health and Human Services. Get ready for grants management. Available at: https://www.hhs.gov/grants/grants/get-ready-for-grants-management/index.html. Accessed December 17, 2017.

25. Grants.gov. Search grants. Available at: https://grants.gov/web/grants/search-grants.html. Accessed December 17, 2017.

26. Foundation Center. Foundation Directory Online. Available at: https://fconline.foundationcenter.org. Accessed August 29, 2017.

27. University of Pittsburgh Office of Research. Basics of federal contracting. Available at: http://www.research.pitt.edu/fcs-basics-federal-contracting. Accessed August 28, 2017.

28. Small Business Innovation Research and Small Business Technology Transfer. Course 1, program basics; tutorial 6, contracts vs grants. Available at: https://www.sbir.gov/tutorials/program-basics/tutorial-6#. Accessed August 28, 2017.

29. Centers for Disease Control and Prevention. Funding contracts. Available at: https://www.cdc.gov/contracts/index.html. Accessed August 28, 2017.

30. Maternal and Child Health Bureau, Health Resources and Services Administration. Explore the Title V Federal–State Partnership. Available at: https://mchb.tvisdata.hrsa.gov/Home. Accessed January 25, 2018.

31. Schell S, Luke D, Schooley M, et al. Public health program capacity for sustainability: a new framework. *Implement Sci.* 2013; 8:15.

32. Luke DA, Calhoun A, Robichaux CB, Elliott MB, Moreland-Russell S. The program sustainability assessment tool: a new instrument for public health programs. *Prev Chronic Dis.* 2014; 11:130184.

33. Minyard K, Matrinez A, Adimu T. Position for sustainability. In: Michener JL, Koo D, Castrucci BC, Sprague JB, eds. *The Practical Playbook.* New York, NY: Oxford Press; 2016:83–94.

34. Center for Public Health Systems Science. The Program Sustainability Assessment Tool. Washington University in St Louis. 2012. Available at: https://sustaintool.org. Accessed January 4, 2018.

35. Georgia Health Policy Center. Sustainability Formative Assessment Tool. 2011. Available at: https://www.ruralhealthinfo.org/sustainability/pdf/sustainability-self-assessment-tool.pdf. Accessed January 4, 2018.

36. Tuckman BW. Development sequence in small groups. *Psychol Bull.* 1965;63(6):384–399.

37. Scholtes P, Joiner B, Streibel B. *The Team Handbook.* 3rd ed. Madison, WI: Oriel Incorporated; 2003.

38. Goal/QPC. *The Team Memory Jogger.* Madison, WI: Oriel Incorporated; 1995.

39. Brassard M, Ritter D. Team guidelines. In: Brassard M, Ritter D, eds. *The Memory Jogger 2: Tools for Continuous Improvement and Effective Planning.* Salem, NH: Goal/QPC; 2010.

40. Begun JW, Malcolm JK. Drive for execution and continuous improvement in public health programs and organizations. In: Begun JW, Malcolm JK, eds. *Leading Public Health: A Competency Framework.* New York, NY: Springer Publishing Company; 2014.

41. Mosser G, Begun J. Evaluating healthcare teams and team members. In: Mosser G, Begun JW, eds. *Understanding Teamwork in Health Care.* New York, NY: McGraw-Hill; 2014.

42. De Oliveira J. How to have difficult conversations. In: Michener JL, Koo D, Castrucci BC, Sprague JB, eds. *The Practical Playbook.* New York, NY: Oxford Press; 2016:65–68.

43. Public Health Foundation. Quality improvement in public health. Available at: http://www.phf.org/focusareas/qualityimprovement/Pages/Quality_Improvement.aspx. Accessed January 18, 2018.

44. Public Health Foundation. When to apply QI tools to support measurement activities. Available at: http://www.phf.org/resourcestools/Documents/QI%20Tools%20and%20Measurement%20Activities.pdf. Accessed January 18, 2019.

45. Minnesota Department of Health. PDSA: Plan-do-study-act. Available at: http://www.health. state.mn.us/divs/opi/qi/toolbox/pdsa.html. Accessed January 18, 2018.

46. Project Management Institute. Who are project managers? Available at: https://www.pmi.org/ about/learn-about-pmi/who-are-project-managers. Accessed February 16, 2018.

47. Scholtes P. *The Leader's Handbook. Making Things Happen, Getting Things Done.* New York, NY: McGraw-Hill; 1998.

48. Project Management Institute. Available at: https://www.pmi.org. Accessed February 16, 2018.

49. Collaboration for Impact. The backbone organisation. Available at: http://www.collaboration forimpact.com/collective-impact/the-backbone-organisation. Accessed February 16, 2018.

50. Turner S, Merchant K, Kania J, Martin E. Understanding the value of backbone organizations in collective impact: part 2. Stanford University. 2012. *Stanford Social Innovation Review.* Available at: https://ssir.org/articles/entry/understanding_the_value_of_backbone_organizations_in_ collective_impact_2. Accessed February 16, 2018.

9

Policy in Public Health

Barbara Langland-Orban, PhD, and Jacqueline Wiltshire, PhD

INTRODUCTION

Policy development is one of three core public health functions, the other two being **assessment** and **assurance**. In the United States, public health policies are developed at federal, state, and local levels. Centers for Disease Control and Prevention (**CDC**) defines policy as "a law, regulation, procedure, administrative action, incentive, or voluntary practice of governments and other institutions." The health of our nation is influenced by public health policies—examples include tobacco control policies and school nutrition policies for healthier meals in schools.[1] Thus, public health policy can take many forms to advance the public's health, from creating incentives to outright mandates. For example, states can use cigarette sales taxes as an incentive to reduce smoking via the added expense or, alternatively, can ban smoking in public places or restaurants, thereby prohibiting smoking in these places while also precluding exposure to secondhand smoke.

The **10 Essential Public Health Services** identify public health activities that are relevant to all communities. Three of the services are associated with the policy development public health function[2]:

1. Inform, educate, and empower people about health issues.
2. Mobilize community partnerships and action to identify and solve health problems.
3. Develop policies and plans that support individual and community health efforts.[2]

This chapter provides an overview of public health policy in the United States by addressing the following 14 tasks:

- ❑ Develop positions on health issues, law, and policy.
- ❑ Establish goals, timelines, funding alternatives, or partnership opportunities for influencing policy initiatives.
- ❑ Defend existing health policies, programs, and resources.
- ❑ Educate policy- and decision-makers to improve health, social justice, and equity.
- ❑ Use scientific evidence, best practices, stakeholder input, or public opinion data to inform policy and program decision-making.
- ❑ Assess positions of key stakeholders for health policies, programs, and resources.
- ❑ Promote the adoption of health policies, programs, and resources.

❑ Identify the social and economic impact of a health policy, program, or initiative.
❑ Analyze political, social, and economic policies that affect health systems at the local, national, or global levels.
❑ Measure changes in health systems (including input, processes, and output).
❑ Determine the feasibility and expected outcomes of policy options (e.g., health, fiscal, administrative, legal, ethical, social, political).
❑ Analyze policy options when designing programs.
❑ Ensure the consistency of policy integration into organizational plans, procedures, structures, and programs.
❑ Implement federal, state, or local regulatory programs and guidelines.

MAJOR CONTENT

Develop Positions on Health Issues, Law, and Policy

The **policymaking process** begins with recognizing a problem in which discontent exists with the status quo among the general public, advocacy groups, special interests, and/or policymakers. The "problem" becomes the target for the policymaking process, which has six general phases[3]:

1. **Agenda setting** is key in the policy process and pertains to getting the problem on the agenda whereby Congress, state legislators, or local public officials seek to address the identified problem.
2. **Policy formulation** is when policies are proposed to address the problem and then debated by policymakers. Although policymakers may agree a problem is important, inaction can occur if an acceptable policy solution is not agreed upon.
3. **Policy adoption** occurs through established governmental processes in which laws or ordinances are passed by lawmakers.
4. **Policy implementation** occurs after a policy is adopted when government units make the policy operational, which requires both human and financial resources.
5. **Policy evaluation** follows implementation to determine whether the policy is meeting its goals in addressing the identified problem.
6. **Policy modification** occurs after policy evaluation when results are used to determine if a policy should be continued, modified, or repealed.

Please note that some typologies for the policymaking process may have fewer or more steps, which occurs from collapsing activities into a single step or expanding one of the steps into two or more.

John Kingdon is a political scientist who theorized that a policy "**window of opportunity**" occurs when three factors ("**streams of activity**") are present that can lead to policy change. The first is strong support among the voting public and policymakers that a problem should be resolved, which is consistent with the first step of the policymaking process. The second is support for the proposed policy design, which is consistent with the second step of the policymaking process. The third factor is political relationships that are receptive to change.[4]

Vignette 1: *Title XVIII of the Social Security Act (Medicare) was enacted in 1965 under President Lyndon Johnson. In general, Medicare provides health care coverage to persons who are 65 years and older. It was later expanded to also cover younger persons who qualify for Social Security disability benefits or have end-stage renal disease. As passed in 1965, original Medicare included Parts A and B. Parts C and D were added after and are discussed later in this chapter. Medicare Part A covers hospital inpatient care and is funded by a payroll tax that is paid by both employers and employees. Medicare Part B covers supplemental medical (physician and outpatient) services. Participation in Part B requires Medicare beneficiaries to pay a monthly premium that is supplemented (subsidized) by federal funds.*[5]

1. The Medicare policy "window of opportunity" in 1965 was successful with the passage of Medicare because of what factor(s)?
   a. The public perceived that a problem existed.
   b. Support existed for the policy design.
   c. A majority in Congress supported the plan.
   d. All of the above

Answer: d. All of the above factors contributed to its success. As workers retire, they typically lose access to their employer-sponsored health plan. The public and policymakers perceived an issue because older persons had problems purchasing individual private health insurance coverage because of their higher costs from increased likelihood of chronic diseases and hospitalizations. Both Democrats and Republicans supported Medicare, which was a policy solution designed to meet the interests of both political parties. Democrats sought hospital coverage, which was included in Medicare Part A, whereas Republicans sought a federal subsidy for physician coverage, which was included in Medicare Part B. Part B requires a premium, which satisfied fiscally conservative Republicans. Thus, the "window of opportunity" resulted in Medicare passing because consensus existed about the problem and the policy solution, and a favorable political climate existed.

Similar to private health insurance, Medicare Parts A and B were designed to have **cost-sharing** provisions (e.g., deductibles, copayments, and co-insurance), such that beneficiaries share in the cost of services received. This means Medicare recipients can still incur significant expense despite being covered by Medicare. One intent of cost sharing is to avoid **moral hazard** whereby the demand for services increases, in particular unnecessary services, if they are provided at no cost to patients. Thus, Medicare coverage does not cover all *costs* of health services.

Vignette 2: *The **Patient Protection and Affordable Care Act (ACA)** was enacted in 2010. The ACA is also known as "Obamacare" because it is health reform advanced under President Barack Obama. The law is comprehensive, and full implementation regarding private health insurance coverage was implemented on January 1, 2014. A key provision is that employers with 50 or more employees must purchase health insurance for their employees or otherwise pay a penalty. It also required noncovered individuals who do not qualify for Medicaid to purchase health insurance, with federal subsidies to those with qualifying incomes. Individual coverage can be purchased through a state or federal insurance "exchange" where insurance is purchased absent consideration of pre-existing medical conditions.[6] The ACA provisions are somewhat similar to employer-sponsored health insurance in which insurance premiums are based on a group and not an individual's health status or prior use of health services.*

2. The ACA legislation was passed as a result of what factor(s)?
   a. The policy solution was embraced by a majority of Republicans in Congress.
   b. The majority in Congress supported the proposed policy solution.
   c. The political climate between Republicans and Democrats was favorable.
   d. All of the above.

Answer: b. It was passed because the majority in Congress supported the proposed policy solution. This occurred because the majority were Democrats, as was President Obama. Republicans in the House or Senate did not support the ACA. This subsequently resulted in contentious relationships, leading to repeated attempts by some Republicans to repeal the ACA, which did not occur until a policy solution was agreed upon by Congress and President Donald Trump in December 2017 via a tax bill. The law was changed to eliminate the penalty associated with the mandate to purchase health insurance beginning in 2019.[7] This may have an impact on health insurance markets and premiums if healthy individuals choose not to purchase health insurance. Nonetheless, other ACA provisions remain.

The three branches of government (legislative, executive, and judicial) are designed to create a separation of powers to protect citizen rights, and each is involved in the policy-making process. The federal legislative branch (also known as Congress) passes laws, controls spending and tax policy, and holds the power to declare war. The executive branch (led by the president) signs bills into law (or alternatively vetoes them) and is responsible for enforcing laws and regulations through the various federal agencies and departments. In the judicial branch (the courts), laws that are passed can be challenged by states, members of the public, or special interests. The US Constitution recognizes "one supreme Court"—the US Supreme Court, which is committed to preserving and protecting the US Constitution. The Supreme Court decides which cases it will hear based on the constitutional challenges involved. Their judgments are generally final (see Chapter 4, "Law and Ethics," for more information).[8,9]

For a bill to become law, both chambers of Congress (House of Representatives and Senate) must each pass a version of the bill. Bills that raise taxes can only begin in the

House. Once both chambers have passed a version, the two bills are referred to a **conference committee**, which includes key relevant members of the House and Senate, to resolve differences in the two bills. If consensus is achieved, a conference report is sent back to the House and Senate for a vote.[10] If it is passed by both chambers, the president can either sign the bill into law or veto it. If it is vetoed, the bill is sent back to the House and Senate for another vote. Overriding a President's veto requires a two-thirds vote in both the House and Senate, which infrequently occurs.[11]

Establish Goals, Timelines, Funding Alternatives, or Partnership Opportunities for Influencing Policy Initiatives

Similar to Medicare, **Title XIX of the Social Security Act (Medicaid)** was enacted in 1965.[5] Original Medicaid covers low-income persons in special needs categories, such as pregnant women, children, nursing home residents, and the blind and disabled, thereby covering certain vulnerable populations. Medicaid is funded by the federal government along with the state government matching funds. Medicaid is administered by each state, and programs vary by state with some states providing more generous benefits than others. Thus, Medicaid is a federal–state partnership.

Vignette 3: *Medicaid expansion was passed as part of the ACA in 2010 and would require states to expand Medicaid coverage to cover all low-income adults aged 18 to 64 years who were at less than or equal to 138% of the federal poverty level. Each state's expansion was to be implemented on January 1, 2014. Initially, the Medicaid expansion would be funded solely by federal funds and later transition to federal and state matching funds.*

3. Since then, what occurred with the Medicaid expansion?
   a. All states have expanded Medicaid consistent with the ACA.
   b. Some states have requested waivers to avoid the mandate to expand Medicaid.
   c. The US Supreme Court overturned the mandate for states to expand Medicaid.
   d. Some states have been given approval to delay their Medicaid expansion.

Answer: c. In 2012, the US Supreme Court overturned the mandate for states to expand Medicaid, following legal challenges from many states. The court found the mandate "unconstitutionally coercive of states" because states had insufficient notification to voluntarily agree to an expansion, and noncompliance could result in a state losing all federal Medicaid funding.[12] As a consequence, about 18 states have not expanded Medicaid, thereby forgoing federal funds to cover low-income adults. The other answers are not correct regarding approvals and waivers and not all states expanded Medicaid coverage consistent with the ACA.

It should be noted the **US Constitution** establishes the central laws and principles by which the United States is governed. It has been asserted that the Constitution creates challenges to health reform because of some of its provisions.[3]

The **State Children's Health Insurance Program (SCHIP or CHIP) is Title XXI of the Social Security Act** and was enacted in 1997. It covers children who do not qualify for original Medicaid, but whose family incomes are insufficient to afford private health insurance. States are allowed to provide SCHIP funding through Medicaid, through a distinct SCHIP program, or through a combination of Medicaid and a distinct program. In general, the federal–state funding match has been 70% federal and 30% state, which was intended to encourage states to develop the program. To receive the funds, each state must submit a Title XXI plan for approval. Similar to Medicaid, SCHIP programs are administered by each state; however, benefits must achieve certain standards. The program has been successful in enrollment and meeting health care needs among enrolled children.[13–15]

Medicare, Medicaid, and SCHIP are all governed by the federal **Centers for Medicare and Medicaid Services (CMS)**, which provides coverage to more than 100 million persons. The goal of CMS is to cover eligible individuals, as well as to improve quality and affordability of health care for its beneficiaries. CMS is an agency under the **US Department of Health and Human Services (HHS)**. The mission of HHS is "to enhance and protect the well-being of all Americans." Its scope encompasses medicine, social services, and public health. HHS accomplishes its mission though various offices and agencies, which include **CDC**, Food and Drug Administration (**FDA**), National Institutes of Health (**NIH**), Health Resources and Services Administration (**HRSA**), Agency for Healthcare Research and Quality (**AHRQ**), Indian Health Service (**IHS**), Agency for Toxic Substances and Disease Registry (**ATSDR**), Office of Civil Rights (**OCR**), Substance Abuse and Mental Health Services Administration (**SAMHSA**), and many other offices that are described on the HHS Web site.[16,17]

Defend Existing Health Policies, Programs, and Resources

The **Iron Triangle** of health care is **access, quality, and cost**, which are the focus of public health policies, programs, and resources. Access pertains to being able to receive needed services or resources, such as clean water or a clinic visit for a medical problem. Many barriers exist to access, such as geographic, transportation, or financial barriers and personal conflicts (e.g., work). The Institute of Medicine (**IOM**), now known as the National Academy of Medicine (**NAM**), identified six aims to improve health care quality, which are to provide care that is (1) safe, (2) effective, (3) timely, (4) patient-centered, (5) efficient, and (6) equitable.[18] The World Health Organization (**WHO**) has embraced this typology and defines quality as "the extent to which health care services provided to individuals and patient populations improve desired health outcomes. In order to achieve this, health care must be safe, effective, timely, efficient, equitable and people-centered."[19] Cost is focused on affordability, which is a major concern for "ordinary" persons. In the United States, health care is expensive and can result in major medical debt that is difficult, if not impossible, to pay. The current policy dilemma regarding cost is advancing policies that render health care more affordable without creating burdensome regulation.[20] The ACA is an example of public policy designed to make health care and insurance more affordable.

The following vignettes provide examples of how public health policies have been developed to advance access and quality.

Vignette 4: *Joe had the flu and weeks later was not fully recovered. As a consequence, he visited his local emergency department (ED) and reported his chief complaint as acute shortness of breath and said he might have pneumonia. The triage nurse explained that because Joe was uninsured, it was better for him to use the hospital's urgent care center, which was a few blocks away. The nurse explained this would be less costly because an ED visit can result in a large hospital bill of $1,000 or more.*

4. Which federal policy is most relevant to this scenario?
   a. Value-based purchasing
   b. Emergency Medical Treatment and Labor Act
   c. Health Insurance Portability and Accountability Act (HIPAA)
   d. Meaningful use

Answer: b. The scenario presents a violation of the federal **Emergency Medical Treatment and Labor Act (EMTALA)** because an ED screening examination was not provided and, therefore, it is unknown if Joe needed emergency care, such as antibiotics for pneumonia. EMTALA was passed by Congress in 1986 to ensure emergency care is *accessible* to all persons (including the uninsured) and not based on a patient's ability to pay. EMTALA requires hospitals with an ED to provide a medical screening examination when a patient presents to the ED, as well as to treat or stabilize any true emergency, including women in active labor. If the screening examination determines that the condition is not an emergency, EMTALA obligations have been met even if the underlying medical condition still exists.[21] The other choices to this question are not correct as they relate to other policy issues including rewards or penalties for quality of care (a), privacy and security of health information (c), and meaningful use of electronic health records (EHRs; d).

EMTALA is an unfunded mandate, such that hospitals and physicians risk not being paid for the EMTALA services they are required to provide. This results in **cost shifting** in which patients with private insurance may experience higher costs in order to help fund care provided to those who cannot afford to pay.[22] Thus, it is advantageous for communities to have everyone covered by a health plan to avoid cost shifting.

Vignette 5: *Fred, a Medicare beneficiary, also had the flu and subsequently visited the ED for acute shortness of breath. The triage nurse cautioned that his wait could be long as many sick patients were waiting to be seen. Two hours later, Fred was still in the waiting room.*

Following multiple unanswered requests about his status in the queue, Fred notified the triage nurse that he was leaving without being seen because of their slow service.

5. Which federal policy is most relevant to Fred's experience?
   a. Value-based purchasing
   b. Medicare Access and Chip Reauthorization Act (MACRA)
   c. Emergency Medical Treatment & Labor Act
   d. All of the above

Answer: a. The scenario reflects the importance of Medicare's **value-based purchasing** program, which financially rewards or penalizes hospitals according to the *quality* of care provided to Medicare patients. Value-based purchasing was established by the ACA and implemented in 2013. Medicare has developed quality metrics that are used to create incentive payments based on how well a hospital performs *or* how well they improve performance relative to past performance. One ED metric is the percentage of patients who left before being seen, which is included on Medicare's **Hospital Compare** Web site, under the hospital's category for "Timely and Effective Care" (see Emergency Department Care).[23] EMTALA is not relevant because the patient chose to leave before the screening examination. MACRA pertains to physician payments and therefore is not relevant to the scenario.

In addition, the patient experience domain of value-based purchasing uses findings from the national **Hospital Consumer Assessment of Healthcare Providers and Systems (HCAHPS) survey**, which asks hospital patients about their satisfaction with factors such as communication with doctors and nurses, responsiveness of hospital staff, discharge instructions, and overall rating of the hospital. Hospitals with low patient satisfaction ratings can receive lesser reimbursement from Medicare. In addition, Medicare has a **Consumer Assessment of Healthcare Providers and Systems** for other types of providers, including physicians, nursing homes, and home health agencies.[24]

Value-based purchasing is an example of Medicare transitioning from paying solely on the basis of volume of services to also integrating value (quality). Similar to hospitals, physicians and other clinicians are likewise being rewarded for meeting quality metrics, such as through the **Physician Quality Reporting System** and more recently through **MACRA,** which modifies the way physicians can be paid for Medicare patients. MACRA provides a Quality Payment Program that includes two new programs: **Advanced Alternative Payment models** and the **Merit-Based Incentive Payment System**.[25] These are examples of how public health policy is used to improve health care quality for Medicare patients.

The ACA also created the **Center for Medicare and Medicaid Innovation (CMMI)**, also known as the "Innovation Center." It is charged with designing, testing, and implementing new payment models that address enhancing quality, containing costs, and reducing inefficiencies in care delivery. CMMI is testing many new payment models (e.g., for medical homes, accountable care organizations, and bundled payments).[26]

Educate Policy- and Decision-Makers to Improve Health, Social Justice, and Equity

Educating policymakers to improve health, social justice, and equity reflects the "Agenda Setting" step of the policymaking process. Many examples exist of major public policies that reflect efforts to successfully educate policymakers to improve health, social justice, and equity for populations. For example, the **Social Security Act** was passed in 1935 to provide for social welfare, which included guaranteed retirement insurance (Social Security) and public assistance for persons who are unable to work. **Title V of the Social Security Act** was included to advance the health of mothers and children, including children with special needs. Each state administers its Title V program through its state health agency. Title V is funded through a Maternal and Child Health block grant, which is funded annually by Congress. These federal funds must be matched with state or local funds. The **Maternal and Infant Care** program was added to Title V in 1965. Beginning in 2015, states are held accountable to develop a strategic plan that addresses their priorities relative to national outcome measures, national performance measures, and evidence-based strategy measures.[27,28]

Another example is the **Ryan White HIV/AIDS Program,** which provides federal funds for care and support services to underinsured or uninsured patients who have HIV. The Ryan White program provides grant funding to population areas that are severely affected by HIV; to community-based organizations that support early intervention; to family-centered care for infants, children, youth, and women with HIV; and for research and training of providers. The program is an example of how federal funds can be directed to effective organizations or regions with the greatest needs.[29]

In addition, states can use **Section 1115 Medicaid Demonstration Waivers of the Social Security Act** to provide demonstration or pilot projects that are designed to better meet state Medicaid objectives in serving qualified low-income and vulnerable populations. This enhances meeting state-specific priorities to improve health, social justice, and equity. Projects must be approved by the secretary of HHS and be budget-neutral relative to federal funding.[30] For example, 19 states are using Section 1115 waivers to provide enhanced behavioral health services, including services for substance use disorder.[31]

Use Scientific Evidence, Best Practices, Stakeholder Input, or Public Opinion Data to Inform Policy and Program Decision-Making

Numerous data sources exist to identify and document public health problems that need policy solutions. For example, CDC's **National Center for Health Statistics** provides substantive information by program or topic, as well as data, including statistics by state.[32] By topic, data include prevalence, mortality, statistics, and related Web sites, and the topics are diverse, such as chronic disease, environmental health, and life expectancy.[33] Also, the Robert Wood Johnson Foundation and University of Wisconsin have collaborated to create the **County Health Rankings & Roadmaps** Web site, which allows for choosing a state or county to review overall health outcomes and health factors.[34] One limitation of such sources is they do not provide zip code (or within-county) health disparities.

In addition to the sources that identify community health problems, other resources identify evidence-based solutions. For example, *The Guide to Community Preventive Services*, developed by HHS in 1996, provided evidence-based information on various policy interventions relative to their effectiveness and cost by topic area.[35] Similarly, AHRQ's **National Guideline Clearinghouse** provided comparable information regarding clinical practice guidelines by topic area[36]; however, this resource lost federal funding in 2018.

Vignette 6: *Before the 1992 presidential election, Democratic candidate Bill Clinton campaigned for health reform that would provide universal health care coverage. Once elected, President Clinton's health reform plan was titled the* **Health Security Act of 1993**.

6. Clinton's health reform plan primarily failed because of what factor?
   a. The public did not perceive that a problem existed.
   b. The policy solution was not evidence-based and thus not embraced by a majority.
   c. Congress did not appropriate funds for the law after it was passed.
   d. Both Republicans and Democrats in Congress opposed health reform.

Answer: b. The policy problem was clear because of rising health care and health insurance costs, coupled with 37 million uninsured citizens. President Clinton's wife, Hillary Clinton, led the task force to address national health care reform, which was dominated by academicians. The proposed Health Security Act of 1993 would mandate employers to purchase health insurance for all employees. The health insurance industry, a major stakeholder, actively opposed the Act for being too complex and for restricting choice when individuals select a health plan. The industry created advertisements that alerted the public that they may not be able to keep their current health plan, even if satisfied with the plan. Although it was debated in Congress, the Health Security Act never came to a vote in the House or Senate. The proposed policy design had not been previously used, making the outcomes and potential problems unknown. By contrast, the ACA of 2010 was modeled after health reform in the state of Massachusetts, which was successful and effective in significantly reducing the percentage of uninsured persons. This reveals the **importance of having evidence** that a policy solution is effective before broadly implementing it. Untested interventions are better used in demonstration or pilot studies.

Assess Positions of Key Stakeholders for Health Policies, Programs, and Resources

Mobilizing for Action through Planning and Partnerships (MAPP) was developed by CDC and the **National Association of City and County Health Officials** (**NACCHO**) from 1997 to 2000. NACCHO is a professional organization that advocates for 2,800 local health departments throughout the United States. MAPP is used to develop local strategic plans for community health improvement, integrating the 10 Essential Public Health Services and the **National Public Health Performance Standards**. A key part of the MAPP process is engaging community representatives and stakeholders in visioning and priority setting using data (evidence), which are then used to create a strategic plan for a community. Plans include goals, objectives, and needed actions. MAPP is also used by state health agencies and their partners as a statewide improvement process. MAPP provides for identifying actions to problems, some of which require public policy solutions.[37-41]

The National Public Health Performance Standards program provides tools for a "Local Public Health Assessment" and a "Public Health Governing Entity Assessment." The findings of these assessments are integrated into the MAPP process. In addition, a "State Public Health Assessment" tool is available, hosted by the **Association of State and Territorial Health Officials**, with findings similarly integrated into state planning processes and used for advocacy in public health policy.[42]

Vignette 7: *For 40 years, the Merryville County Health Department has actively engaged in community public health planning. They have consistently used the most current public health planning tools available to them.*

7. Before using MAPP, which public health planning tool would Merryville County Health Department have used?
   a. Planned Approach to Community Health
   b. Assessment Protocol for Excellence in Public Health
   c. IOM Model
   d. All of the above

Answer: d. In 1985, CDC created the planning tool **Planned Approach to Community Health,** which provided a procedure for analyzing health problems and their root causes to plan actions that address the problem. In 1991, the **Assessment Protocol for Excellence in Public Health** was developed by NACCHO, in partnership with CDC. It provides self-assessment tools for public health agencies, which include internal and external capacity assessments. The IOM had an expert panel review the various community health assessment models and recommended an **IOM model**, which was published in 1997. It focuses on forming community coalitions to identify and prioritize health problems and subsequently develop, implement, and monitor intervention strategies.[40] MAPP was subsequently developed. All of these processes were used to identify problems and solutions, with some solutions indicating the need for public policy change (see Chapter 6, "Collaboration and Partnership," and Chapter 7, "Program Planning and Evaluation," for more information).

Promote the Adoption of Health Policies, Programs, and Resources

Influencing the adoption of health policies, programs, and resources is accomplished through numerous approaches. These include advocacy, lobbying, campaign fundraising, political action committees, research studies that create evidence, and use of the media.

Advocacy occurs at local, state, and federal levels and is central in advancing public health goals. Advocacy can be done by "ordinary citizens" who write letters (e-mail) or meet with public officials or their staff to influence perspectives on particular health issues or goals. Advocacy techniques include testifying before a city council, a county or a state legislative committee, or a Congressional committee on a health issue to educate decision-makers. Such oral presentations are often accompanied with written testimony to the council or the committee.[10]

By contrast, **lobbying** focuses on communication with policymakers and/or their staff about a particular ordinance, regulation, or law under consideration. Communication can be written or oral to encourage a vote or action for or against the proposed policy. All lobbying encompasses advocacy, but not all advocacy is lobbying. Grass roots lobbying occurs by encouraging members of the public or a professional association or organization to contact policymakers about a particular policy under consideration to take a particular action.[43]

Lobbying and advocacy are often well organized by professional associations, such as the National Rifle Association. In public health, the **American Public Health Association (APHA)** works with its members and state affiliates to address current public health concerns. Their advocacy Web site recommends taking action on issues, such as signing a petition to the president to continue the benefits achieved by the ACA. They also provide "Action Alerts" that encourage members to communicate with policymakers on specific legislation, such as protecting the Clean Air Act. Furthermore, the APHA has a Public Health Action Campaign that provides a tool set to influence public policy decisions (e.g., attending public meetings, writing an op-ed for publication in a newspaper).[44] Similarly, NACCHO advocates for the role of local health departments in assuring communities are safe and healthy.[45]

Nonprofit organizations and professional associations are allowed to engage in lobbying. However, the Internal Revenue Service restricts the amount of their budget that can be used for lobbying. Also, nonprofits are prohibited from using federal funds for lobbying.[46]

Vignette 8: *Following clinical trials, a pharmaceutical company hired a firm to advance the approval of its new drug through the FDA.*

8. Which of the following means of influence does this best represent?
   a. Grass roots lobbying
   b. Political Action Committee (PAC)
   c. Political fundraising
   d. Lobbyist

Answer: d. **Registered lobbyists** are hired to influence public policy, including regulators. They are paid professionals who represent one or more interest groups, such as an organization, association, or industry (e.g., the American Medical Association [AMA]). All states require paid lobbyists to register. Each state is responsible for identifying who is required to register, typically based on compensation received. While "lobbying" per se reflects a citizen's right to free speech, lobbying that is conducted by paid professionals who influence government policies on behalf of an organization or interest group is governed by states.[47,48] Grass roots lobbying is an incorrect response, as there was no attempt to get people to contact the FDA in support of the drug. There was no PAC or fundraising, so these responses are likewise incorrect.

Similar to advocacy, registered lobbyists meet with public officials and their staff on issues of interest, while focused on being persuasive to gain support from policymakers, such as providing research results. They need to provide information that will allow policymakers to explain their support for a policy, program, or resource.[49] In 2015, the health-related organizations that spent the most money on lobbying at the federal level were the AMA, the Pharmaceutical Research and Manufacturers of America, the American Hospital Association, Pfizer, CVS Health, AmGen, Eli Lilly & Co., and the America's Health Insurance Plans.[50]

In addition, campaign fundraising can be used to influence policymakers, as candidates receive funds from individuals and/or special interests to help finance their campaign. However, such contributions do not guarantee how a policymaker will vote on a particular issue. In addition, **PACs** are fundraising entities that exist to generate funds to advance specific issues, candidates, or political parties. Also, the news media has an important role in framing policy issues and providing relevant data and information, including opinion polls.[51] Thus, many alternatives exist to influence public health policy, including advocacy, lobbying, financial contributions, research (evidence), and the media.

Another approach to promoting the adoption of public policy is through **earmarks**. Each year, members of Congress submit their list of special or local projects they seek to have funded to their appropriations committee. The projects may represent requests from individuals, organizations, or state governments. A uniqueness to an earmark is that it is specific to a particular entity when inserted into an appropriations bill, such as a particular organization or location, meaning it is not competitive. State legislatures can likewise use earmarks to fund projects in specific locations. **Appropriation bills** determine the level of spending for such.[10]

Identify the Social and Economic Impact of a Health Policy, Program, or Initiative

Many types of evaluation methods can be used to assess the economic impact of a policy or program (see Chapter 8, "Program Management," for more information on these evaluation concepts)[52]:

- **Cost analyses** measure costs (direct and indirect) absent consideration of benefits.
- **Cost minimization analyses** are used to compare two different interventions relative to the intended outcome. A drawback of this approach is that interventions often produce different outcomes, such that another method is needed.

- **Cost-effectiveness analyses (CEA)** are commonly used when outcomes of interventions differ. They quantify all costs and outcomes to compare alternative interventions by measuring the change in "cost per unit change in effect."
- **Cost–utility analyses** are similar to CEA, but with outcomes measured as some form of health utility, such as quality of life. **Quality of life measures** typically require patient surveys that gauge physical and mental health, as well as social functioning.
- **Cost–benefit analyses** use dollars to measure both costs and benefits. Thus, it estimates the dollar amount of benefits relative to costs. This allows programs to be compared on the basis of their benefit-to-cost ratio.

Analyze Political, Social, and Economic Policies That Affect Health Systems at the Local, National, or Global Levels

Government enactments (i.e., laws, regulations, executive orders, and judicial decisions) are designed to affect the well-being of a population function within interconnected social and economic contexts.[53,54] American health policymaking involves various institutions and actors with opposing views and interest; thus, any policy designed to affect the health system has a political context.[4,53]

An example of a highly political social policy is the 1973 judicial decision making abortion legal in the United States. Depending on political leaning of the Executive and Legislative branches, the federal government has restricted or loosened funding requirements for national programs or organizations that provide reproductive services for women.[55] For example, the Hyde Amendment (which bans the use of federal funds for abortion except in cases to save the woman's life or pregnancy resulting from incest or rape) restricts abortion coverage for people insured by Medicaid or Medicare.[56] States have also restricted access to abortions through technicality and regulation. For example, some states require that women receive counseling and/or wait a specified amount of time before an abortion is performed.[57] Other states require that an ultrasound be part of the abortion service provision.[58] Some states require doctors who perform abortions to have admitting privileges at a local hospital, although there is no medical basis or public health justification for this. Thus, financing and regulatory requirements have an impact on the ability of health systems to provide comprehensive reproductive health care services for women.[59,60]

Addressing climate change is considered the greatest global health challenge of the 21st century.[61] Extreme weather events (floods, heat waves, drought, severe storms) have an impact on population health through air pollution, food and water insecurity, forced migration and displacement, the spread of communicable diseases, and mental health burdens.[61,62] Governments and health systems must have mitigation and adaptation strategies or policies to address the health consequences of climate change.[62] However, US climate change policy is a polarizing political issue.[63] In December 2015, representatives from 195 countries signed a global policy framework (known as the Paris Agreement) to adopt green energy sources, cut down on climate change emissions, and limit the rise of global temperatures.[64] In June 2017, the United States announced that it will withdraw from the Paris Agreement, a controversial decision made by the executive branch of the government. There have also been rollbacks on federal policies and programs on climate change. Cities, states, and businesses that account for more than 50% of the US economy have decided to pledge their commitment to the Paris Agreement; however, nonfederal policies cannot replace federal climate action.[64] The shift in federal policy indicates low perceived risks and uncertainties about climate change and undercuts adaptation strategies that the US public health system and medical care system need to respond to climate change.[65]

Vignette 9: *The 2017 Atlantic hurricane season was one of the most destructive hurricane seasons on record. Hurricanes Harvey, Irma, and Maria changed parts of Texas, Florida, and the Caribbean forever. Miami and Tampa, Florida, evacuated populations because of rising sea levels and flooding. Public health and medical care systems faced critical shortages of food and medicine, and thousands of victims with life-threatening injuries and illnesses were left stranded.*[66]

9. Which of the following is most important to address in climate change policy in terms of its impact on population health and health systems?
   a. Economic factors
   b. Political factors
   c. Scientific factors
   d. Global factors
   e. All of the above

Answer: a. Climate change and global warming are largely driven by economic activities and population growth.[63] Political factors (b) is incorrect. There is said to be global consensus that climate change is a major problem and the Paris Agreement is an indication of this understanding among the world's nations to address climate change.[65] Scientific factors (c) is incorrect. Although robust scientific knowledge and analyses are critical in informing choices to address climate change and consequences, scientists have understood for more than a century that human use of fossil fuels would lead to increases in the earth's temperature.[62] Global factors (d) is incorrect. Climate change has a global impact, but "global factors" is an unspecified catch-all phrase.

Measure Changes in Health Systems Using Inputs, Processes, and Outputs

Inputs, processes, and outputs are the foundation for systems theory (see Chapter 6, "Collaboration and Partnership," and Chapter 7, "Program Planning and Evaluation," for more information).

One public policy initiative that increased inputs in an attempt to improve health processes and outcomes (outputs) was the **Hospital Survey and Reconstruction Act** of 1946, also known as the **Hill–Burton Act**. The Hill–Burton Act was intended to fund uncompensated or reduced fee hospital services to the uninsured and underinsured.[67] The law focused on providing post–World War II funding for hospital construction to states that had fewer than 4.5 beds per 1,000 population for the purpose of providing access to communities that otherwise could not afford the cost of a hospital. Although the 4.5 beds per 1,000 population ratio was intended to be a maximum, it subsequently became a goal for some communities. From 1947 to 1971, Hill–Burton provided about 30% of funding for all hospital projects. Although Hill–Burton was modified in 1954 to allow for funding ambulatory and long-term-care facilities, ultimately 75% of funding was invested in hospital construction.[5] Thus, the federal funds were used to create or expand hospitals (inputs) for the purpose of access to hospitalizations (process) that were intended to improve health outcomes (outputs).

However, in 1959, it was recognized that hospital bed availability was used to the extent beds are available, which is known as **Roemer's law** (after Milton Roemer, MD)—a built bed is a filled bed. As a consequence, it was understood that restricting health care capital expenditures in a community was a means to control costs, such as by restricting the expansion of hospital beds.[5] This reflects an understanding of **supplier-induced demand**, whereby suppliers (hospitals and physicians) can use their knowledge and influence to increase demand among consumers (patients). Nonetheless, in 2016, hospitals remained the largest category of US health expenditures at 32%, followed by physicians and clinical services at 20%.[68]

While the initial Hill–Burton Act focused on building hospitals (inputs), the **Regional Medical Programs (RMPs)** legislation was passed in 1965 to focus on heart disease, cancer, and stroke (outcomes). It provided funds (inputs) to develop regional networks of medical schools, academic health centers, and research institutions to focus on patient care (processes) to reduce these three leading causes of death (outcomes). Subsequently, 56 regions were developed. By 1974, RMPs were no longer allocated funds, being replaced by the National Health Planning and Resource Development Act of 1974. By 1976, RMPs were discontinued.[69]

In addition to RMPs, the **Comprehensive Health Planning Act of 1966** had transitioned funding from state categorical grants to block grants (inputs) that gave states enhanced flexibility to meet their public health priorities (processes and outcomes). The Act required statewide planning as block grant programs must adhere to state plans in order to be approved by the Surgeon General. The Act intended to transfer the focus from hospitals to comprehensive health care.[70] This Act likewise was replaced by the National Health Planning and Resource Development Act of 1974.

The **National Health Planning and Resource Development Act of 1974** expanded the government's role in health planning. It required local health system agencies (**HSAs**) to develop detailed health plans for their community focused on health services, but not health outcomes.[40] The HSAs did not have decision-making authority, but instead made recommendations to the state. All states were required to enact **certificate of need (CON)** laws that regulated capital expenditures of hospitals, as well as nursing homes. The law was eventually repealed and the requirement for CON is now optional among states.[71]

More recently, the **Health Information Technology for Economic and Clinical Health Act of 2009** advanced the adoption and use of **EHRs**, including **meaningful use** of health information technology. The Act provided funds (inputs) to hospitals and health professionals to adopt EHR systems to improve clinical decision support and exchange of health information.[72] Providers have received funding for meeting meaningful use objectives. Meaningful use of EHRs was advanced in three stages to improve quality and patient safety. Stage 1 was to advance data capture and sharing, stage 2 was to advance clinical processes, and stage 3 was to advance outcomes, which is still pending implementation.[73] For example, meaningful use objectives include **computerized physician order entry**, which allows for more accurate prescriptions relative to nurses or pharmacists interpreting a physician's handwriting. Also, an EHR can provide an alert if a dosage is outside of the recommended range or is contraindicated by another medication that has been prescribed, thereby having the potential to improve processes and outcomes.

Determine the Feasibility and Expected Outcomes of Policy Options

A major debate in the United States is who produces better outcomes—government or the free market. For example, some politicians advocate the privatization of Medicare in which beneficiaries would receive vouchers toward purchasing a private health plan. By contrast, other politicians advocate Medicare-for-All, which would allow all citizens to have access to Medicare, albeit with funding via payroll taxes and cost sharing, as currently exists.

Medicare Part C allows beneficiaries to choose a **Medicare Advantage** health plan from a list of private managed care plans, such as a health maintenance organization (HMO) or preferred provider organization (PPO). Medicare pays the private plan a fixed monthly amount (capitation rate) to provide an enrollee's Part A and Part B services. Some Medicare Advantage plans provide more extensive Part B services, such as vision or dental care, and some also include prescription drug coverage (Medicare Part D), which is explained in the next paragraph. The Medicare Advantage plan is then responsible for providing all guaranteed services for the fixed capitation rate, meaning the health plan is at risk for losing money based on the services needed by its enrollees. This creates an incentive to avoid unnecessary services, as well as to recruit healthy elderly persons to the plan. Similar to all managed care plans, Medicare Advantage plans have a defined provider network (hospitals and physicians), which reduces provider choice for enrollees because of the cost of receiving care outside of the network. In addition, Medicare Advantage plans have different out-of-pocket costs and different rules for accessing physician specialists. These private Medicare insurance plans have existed since the 1980s, and 20% of Medicare beneficiaries are enrolled in them.[22,74]

Medicare Part D was created through the **Medicare Modernization Act of 2003** and added prescription drug coverage for Medicare beneficiaries beginning in 2006. However, instead of Medicare creating a formulary and using its federal purchasing power to negotiate drug discounts, the law provided for funding private drug benefit plans, meaning Part D coverage is privatized, but subsidized by federal funds. Medicare beneficiaries choose among drug plans that have differing formularies and premiums. The benefit has a deductible and then cost sharing once the deductible is met. The original Part D required Medicare beneficiaries to pay 100% of drug costs between $2,500 and $5,100, which is referred to as the "donut hole."[22] The donut hole was included in the 2003 legislation to contain federal costs for the Part D program. The ACA included provisions to reduce patient costs while in the donut hole from paying 100% of costs to 25% by 2020.[75]

The **Veterans Health Administration (VHA)** is a government-run health system for eligible veterans. It is part of the **US Department of Veterans Affairs (VA)** and has defined benefits, hospitals, and clinics and expertise in areas specific to veterans' needs, such as mental health services. In addition, the VA has an Office of Research and Development to improve veterans' lives, which includes health.[76] The VHA provides an example of government-run health services that offer comprehensive care. The **Veterans Access, Choice, and Accountability Act of 2014** was created to enhance access and quality of care to eligible veterans. It provides the **Veterans Choice Program,** which allows eligible veterans to use community practitioners. Examples of eligibility criteria include having to wait more than 30 days for an appointment or living more than 40 miles from a VA facility. Thus, the VA now offers a private-sector alternative to eligible veterans.[77-79]

TRICARE is a program that provides health plans to uniformed service members and their families through the **Defense Health Agency**, which is part of the **Military Health System**. TRICARE provides different health plans that achieve or exceed the minimum benefits required by the ACA. Depending on the plan, there may be premiums and cost sharing, such as deductibles and copayments. Enrollees may still receive care from a military hospital or clinic if space permits. TRICARE operates similar to a managed care plan in which each region's administration ensures access to a network of private providers.[80]

Analyze Policy Options When Designing Programs

Models, frameworks, and theories (e.g., Data-Driven Policy Analysis Framework or CDC's Policy Analytical Framework) guide policy options or choices to address public health problems.[81,82] Data and policy priorities influence policy options when one is designing a program.[83] The most useful policy is generally based on data or factual information. However, given changing problems and situations in public health problems, policy options are also considered without data or facts. Policy options are generally analyzed in terms of their impact and intended or unintended consequences.[82] These analyses typically consider public health impact (e.g., potential to have an impact on risk factors, disparities, morbidity, and mortality), feasibility (i.e., likelihood of being successfully implemented), and economic or budgetary impact (i.e., costs and benefits).[81,83] Analyzing policies in terms of their impacts and consequences can include before-and-after comparisons of a policy, with-and-without comparisons of a policy, and actual-versus-planned comparisons of a policy on affected individuals, groups, or organizations.[4]

Congress has an infrastructure for gaining information about proposed and existing public health policies and programs. The **Congressional Budget Office** analyses the impact of proposed and current policies on federal costs. The **Government Accountability Office (GAO)** provides an investigative function for Congress. It is independent and nonpartisan and provides fact-based information to Congress, including financial auditing of federal agencies, as well as program evaluations and policy analyses. For example, the GAO's Web site identifies "key issues," such as "duplication and cost savings" to identify areas where efficiencies or cost savings can be achieved. Finally, the **Congressional Research Service** provides comprehensive legislative and policy research to members of Congress.[84,85] Similarly, states establish processes for estimating costs and benefits of proposed and existing public policies, conducting program evaluations, and auditing state agencies.

Ensure the Consistency of Policy Integration Into Organizational Plans, Procedures, Structures, and Programs

Policy integration into plans, procedures, structures, and programs requires **financial resources,** which are secured through the annual budget process. The federal fiscal year is October 1 to September 30; however, states may use a different fiscal year, such as July 1 to June 30.

With the **federal budget,** "the US Constitution grants the 'power of the purse' to Congress."[10] Each year, Congress must develop the budget for the subsequent fiscal year, recognizing that the federal government receives its money from taxes and borrowing. Then, it spends money on (1) mandatory programs (e.g., Medicare and Social Security), (2) paying interest on debt, and (3) discretionary spending. The first step in the federal budget process is for federal agencies and departments to develop and submit their proposals to the White House, in recognition that these agencies and departments report to the president. Then, the president submits his/her budget proposal to Congress, usually by the first Monday in February, which is nearly eight months before the new fiscal year will begin on October 1. Subsequently, both the House and Senate review the president's proposal and each develops a budget resolution regarding overall spending. A conference committee is used to resolve differences between the two budgets. Subsequently, for discretionary spending, the House and Senate appropriations committees divide the budget among 12 subcommittees, which represent the relevant agencies, to then develop appropriations bills. The appropriations bills are voted on by the House and Senate, with conference committees used to resolve differences. Once both chambers vote to support the same bill, it is sent to the president for signature. Congress can pass an **omnibus appropriations bill** if agreement is not reached on the subcommittee appropriations bills, which provides funding for multiple areas. If an appropriations bill is not signed by September 30, the federal government will not have a budget and nonessential services will cease to be provided.[86]

The House and Senate each have committees and subcommittees. The key committees that deal with legislative issues important for health care in the United States are the following:

- The **Senate Health, Education, Labor, and Pensions Committee** has broad jurisdiction or authority over health care, education, labor and retirement policies, and public welfare, including jurisdiction over most HHS agencies and institutes.
- The **Senate Finance Committee** has jurisdiction over taxation and other revenue-related affairs. It is one of the most powerful committees in Congress with jurisdiction over health programs under the Social Security Act, including Medicare, Medicaid, and CHIP.[4]
- The **Senate Committee on Appropriations** is the largest committee in the US Senate. It is responsible for legislation that allocates federal funds to government programs, agencies, and organizations. Its role is defined by the US Constitution.[87]
- The **House Ways and Means Committee** has jurisdiction over all taxation, tariffs, and other revenue-raising measures in the United States.[88] It is one of the most influential committees in the Congress because of its power to tax. Its role is similar to that of the Senate Finance Committee.
- The **House Energy and Commerce Committee (HECC)** has oversight over all the nation's laws ranging from telecommunications to health care. It has the authority to evaluate laws and the agencies that implement them. The HECC also has jurisdiction over Medicaid.[4,89]

Implement Federal, State, or Local Regulatory Programs and Guidelines

Federal regulations are enforced by the relevant federal agency. For example, the FDA provides oversight for food and drugs, as well as medical devices, radiation-emitting products, drugs and food for animals, tobacco, and cosmetics. As an example of enforcement, the FDA works to achieve compliance with the Tobacco Control Act of 2009, which prohibits the sale or marketing of tobacco to minors and also requires health warnings on smokeless tobacco. Compliance is achieved through education and training, surveillance, and penalties that can include warning letters, fines, prohibiting tobacco sales, and seizure of assets.[90,91]

State police powers give states the authority to license hospitals and clinicians, including physicians. In addition, police powers allow states to promote the public's health by enacting laws regarding sanitation, vaccination, and air and water quality. Such laws are intended to reduce morbidity and mortality.[92]

Local officials (e.g., municipalities) must abide by federal and state laws and regulations. **Home rule authority** gives local officials the ability to enact ordinances or regulations that are specific to the community, not otherwise prohibited. The ordinances or regulations are autonomous from the state.[93] For example, in Florida, home rule authority allows local officials to decide whether or not to use community water fluoridation because is it neither required nor prohibited by state or federal law.

CONCLUSION

Policymaking is a cyclical, complex process. It requires gaining agreement among policymakers that a problem needs to be addressed, as well as identification of a suitable and feasible policy solution that policymakers will accept. The process can be greatly influenced by politics, as well as by money, as PACs and campaign contributions influence not only who is elected but also whose interests these elected officials represent. Governmental powers (i.e., federal and state constitutions, home rule, and the common law) shape policy. Thus, public health policy is subject to many influences, some of which are not necessarily focused on advancing the public's health. For example, the United States lacks universal health care coverage, which exists in most developed nations. Despite this, in recent decades, Congress and federal government agencies have worked to ensure access to emergency care, to provide greater transparency regarding quality of care, and to improve access to health insurance among those previously not covered.

A key to influencing public health policy is credible evidence that a policy intervention is effective and affordable, which allows the use of advocacy, lobbying, and the media to advance sound public health policies. Nonetheless, some policies are passed absent any evidence of effectiveness. The development of the public health and health care delivery systems has been through a series of incremental policy improvements. However, significant disparities still exist in many areas, such as access to health care, clean air and water, and emergency and disaster preparedness, which ultimately contribute to overall health disparities in the United States.

REFERENCES

1. Centers for Disease Control and Prevention. Public health policy. 2017. Available at: https://www.cdc.gov/stltpublichealth/policy. Accessed February 5, 2018.

2. Centers for Disease Control and Prevention. The public health system & the 10 essential public health services. 2017. Available at: https://www.cdc.gov/stltpublichealth/publichealthservices/essentialhealthservices.html. Accessed February 5, 2018.

3. Harrington C, Estes CL. *Health Policy: Crisis and Reform in the US Health Care Delivery System.* 4th ed. Sudbury, MA: Jones & Bartlett Learning; 2004.

4. Longest BB. *Health Policy Making in the United States.* 6th ed. Chicago, IL: Health Administration Press; 2016.

5. Starr P. *The Social Transformation of American Medicine.* 2nd ed. New York, NY: Basic Books; 1982.

6. Rosenbaum S. The Patient Protection and Affordable Care Act: implications for public health policy and practice. *Public Health Rep.* 2011;126(1):130–135.

7. Henry J. Kaiser Family Foundation. ACA's future. Available at: https://www.kff.org/tag/aca-future. Accessed February 20, 2018.

8. US House of Representatives. Branches of government. Available at: https://www.house.gov/the-house-explained/branches-of-government. Accessed February 20, 2018.

9. Supreme Court of the United States. About the Court: the Court and constitutional interpretation. Available at: https://www.supremecourt.gov/about/constitutional.aspx. Accessed February 20, 2008.

10. Kennan SA. Legislative relations in public health. In: Novick LF, Morrow CB, Mays GP, eds. *Public Health Administration: Principles for Population-Based Management.* 2nd ed. Sudbury, MA: Jones & Bartlett Learning; 2008.

11. US Senate. Glossary term: override of a veto. Available at: https://www.senate.gov/reference/glossary_term/override_of_a_veto.htm. Accessed February 20, 2018.

12. Henry J. Kaiser Family Foundation. A guide to the Supreme Court's decision on the ACA's Medicaid expansion. 2012. Available at: https://www.kff.org/health-reform/issue-brief/a-guide-to-the-supreme-courts-decision. Accessed February 21, 2018.

13. Lambrew JM. The State Children's Health Insurance Program: past, present, and future. The Commonwealth Fund. 2007. Available at: http://www.commonwealthfund.org/publications/fund-reports/2007/feb/the-state-childrens-health-insurance-program--past--present--and-future. Accessed February 21, 2018.

14. Centers for Medicare & Medicaid Services. CHIP state program information. 2018. Available at: https://www.medicaid.gov/chip/state-program-information/index.html. Accessed February 21, 2018.

15. Social Security. TITLE XXI—State Children's Health Insurance Program. Available at: https://www.ssa.gov/OP_Home/ssact/title21/2100.htm. Accessed February 21, 2018.

16. US Department of Health and Human Services. About HHS. 2017. Available at: https://www.hhs.gov/about/index.html. Accessed February 21, 2018.

17. US Department of Health and Human Services. HHS organizational chart. 2017. Available at: https://www.hhs.gov/about/agencies/orgchart/index.html. Accessed February 21, 2018.

18. Agency for Healthcare Research and Quality. The six domains of health care quality. 2016. Available at: https://www.ahrq.gov/professionals/quality-patient-safety/talkingquality/create/sixdomains.html. Accessed February 21, 2018.

19. World Health Organization. What is quality of care and why is it important? 2018. Available at: http://www.who.int/maternal_child_adolescent/topics/quality-of-care/definition/en. Accessed February 21, 2018.

20. Jost T. Affordability: the most urgent health reform issue for ordinary Americans. Health Affairs Blog. February 29, 2016. Available at: https://www.healthaffairs.org/do/10.1377/hblog20160229.053330/full. Accessed February 21, 2018.

21. Centers for Medicare & Medicaid Services. Emergency Medical Treatment & Labor Act (EMTALA). Available at: https://www.cms.gov/Regulations-and-Guidance/Legislation/EMTALA/index.html. Accessed February 21, 2018.

22. Feldstein PJ. *Health Policy Issues: An Economic Perspective.* 5th ed. Chicago, IL: Health Administration Press; 2011.

23. US Centers for Medicare & Medicaid Services. Hospital compare. Available at: https://www.medicare.gov/hospitalcompare/search.html. Accessed February 21, 2018.

24. Agency for Healthcare Research and Quality. About CAHPS. 2016. Available at: https://www.ahrq.gov/cahps/about-cahps/index.html. Accessed February 22, 2018.

25. Centers for Medicare & Medicaid Services. Quality payment program. 2017. https://www.cms.gov/Medicare/Quality-Payment-Program/Quality-Payment-Program.html. Accessed February 22, 2018.

26. Henry J. Kaiser Family Foundation. "What is CMMI?" and 11 other FAQs about the CMS Innovation Center. 2018. Available at: https://www.kff.org/medicare/fact-sheet/what-is-cmmi-and-11-other-faqs-about-the-cms-innovation-center. Accessed April 13, 2018.

27. Social Security. Title V - Grants to States for Maternal and Child Welfare. Available at: https://www.ssa.gov/history/35actv.html. Accessed February 22, 2017.

28. Health Resources & Services Administration, Maternal & Child Health. Title V Maternal and Child Health Services Block Grant Program. Available at: https://mchb.hrsa.gov/maternal-child-health-initiatives/title-v-maternal-and-child-health-services-block-grant-program. Accessed February 25, 2018.

29. Health Resources & Services Administration, Ryan White & Global HIV/AIDS Programs. About the Ryan White HIV/AIDS Program. Available at: https://hab.hrsa.gov/about-ryan-white-hivaids-program/about-ryan-white-hivaids-program. Accessed February 25, 2018.

30. Centers for Medicare & Medicaid Services. About Section 1115 Demonstrations. Available at: https://www.medicaid.gov/medicaid/section-1115-demo/about-1115/index.html. Accessed February 25, 2018.

31. Henry J. Kaiser Family Foundation. Section 1115 Medicaid Demonstration Waivers: the current landscape of approved and pending waivers. Available at: https://www.kff.org/medicaid/issue-brief/section-1115-medicaid-demonstration-waivers-the-current-landscape-of-approved-and-pending-waivers. Accessed April 14, 2018.

32. Centers for Disease Control and Prevention. National Center for Health Statistics. 2018. Available at: https://www.cdc.gov/nchs/index.htm. Accessed February 25, 2018.

33. Centers for Disease Control and Prevention. Data and statistics. 2018. Available at: https://www.cdc.gov/DataStatistics. Accessed February 25, 2018.

34. County Health Rankings & Roadmaps. How healthy is your community? Available at: http://www.countyhealthrankings.org. Accessed February 25, 2018.

35. US Department of Health and Human Services. About *The Community Guide*. Available at: https://www.thecommunityguide.org/about/about-community-guide. Accessed February 25, 2018.

36. Agency for Healthcare Research and Quality. National Guideline Clearinghouse. Available at: https://www.ahrq.gov/cpi/about/otherwebsites/guideline.gov/index.html. Accessed February 25, 2018.

37. National Association of County and City Health Officials. Your health department's biggest advocate. Available at: https://www.naccho.org/about. Accessed February 25, 2018.

38. National Association of County and City Health Officials. Mobilizing for Action through Planning and Partnerships (MAPP). Available at: https://www.naccho.org/programs/public-health-infrastructure/performance-improvement/community-health-assessment/mapp. Accessed February 25, 2018.

39. National Association of County and City Health Officials. MAPP basics: introduction to the MAPP process. Available at: http://archived.naccho.org/topics/infrastructure/mapp/framework/mappbasics.cfm. Accessed February 25, 2018.

40. Novick LF, Morrow CB, Mays, GP. Assessment and strategic planning in public health. In: Novick LF, Morrow CB, Mays GP, eds. *Public Health Administration: Principles for Population-Based Management*. 2nd ed. Sudbury, MA: Jones & Bartlett Learning; 2008.

41. Hatcher MT, Nicola RM. Engaging communities and building constituencies for public health. In: Shi L, Johnson JA, eds. *Novick & Morrow's Public Health Administration: Principles for Population-Based Management*. 3rd ed. Burlington, MA: Jones & Bartlett Learning; 2014:406.

42. Centers for Disease Control and Prevention. National Public Health Performance Standards. 2017. Available at: https://www.cdc.gov/stltpublichealth/nphps/index.html. Accessed February 26, 2018.

43. National Association of County and City Health Officials. Building your advocacy toolbox: advocacy vs. lobbying. 2016. Available at: https://www.naccho.org/uploads/downloadable-resources/flyer_advocacy-na16-002.pdf. Accessed February 26, 2018.

44. American Public Health Association. Advocacy for public health. 2018. Available at: https://www.apha.org/policies-and-advocacy/advocacy-for-public-health. Accessed February 26, 2018.

45. National Association of County and City Health Officials. Our leadership. Available at: https://www.naccho.org/about/chief-executive-officer-lori-tremmel-freeman-mba. Accessed June 21, 2018.

46. National Council on Aging. Nonprofit advocacy rules & regulations. 2018. Available at: https://www.ncoa.org/public-policy-action/advocacy-toolkit/advocacy-basics/nonprofit-advocacy-rules-regulations. Accessed February 26, 2018.

47. National Conference of State Legislatures. Lobbyist regulation. Available at: http://www.ncsl.org/research/ethics/lobbyist-regulation.aspx. Accessed February 26, 2018.

48. National Conference of State Legislatures. Lobbyist registration requirements. 2017. Available at: http://www.ncsl.org/research/ethics/50-state-chart-lobbyist-registration-requirements.aspx. Accessed February 26, 2018.

49. Weissert CS, Weissert WG. *Governing Health: The Politics of Health Policy*. Baltimore, MD: The Johns Hopkins University Press; 1996:116–117.

50. Rappleye E. Top 20 healthcare lobbyists by spending. August 21, 2015. *Becker's Hospital CFO Report*. Available at: https://www.beckershospitalreview.com/finance/top-20-healthcare-lobbyists-by-spending.html. Accessed February 26, 2018.

51. McLaughlin CP, McLaughlin CD. *Health Policy Analysis: An Interdisciplinary Approach*. Sudbury, MA: Jones & Bartlett Learning; 2008:254–255,262–264.

52. Stoto MA, Cosler LE. Evaluation of public health interventions. In: Novick LF, Morrow CB, Mays GP. *Public Health Administration: Principles for Population-Based Management*. 2nd ed. Sudbury, MA; Jones & Bartlett Learning; 2008:502–508.

53. Herrick JM. Social policy: overview. In: Franklin C, ed. *Encyclopedia of Social Work*. National Association of Social Workers Press, Oxford University Press. 2013.

54. Osypuk TL, Joshi P, Geronimo K, Acevedo-Garcia D. Do social and economic policies influence health? A review. *Curr Epidemiol Rep*. 2014;1(3):149–164.

55. Blendon RJ, Benson JM, Casey LS. Health care in the 2016 election—a view through voters' polarized lenses. *N Engl J Med*. 2016;375(17):e37.

56. Adashi EY, Occhiogrosso RH. The Hyde Amendment at 40 years and reproductive rights in the United States: perennial and panoptic. *JAMA*. 2017;317(15):1523–1524.

57. Kreitzer RJ. Politics and morality in state abortion policy. *State Polit Policy Q.* 2015;15(1): 41–66.

58. Kimport K, Weitz TA. Constructing the meaning of ultrasound viewing in abortion care. *Sociol Health Illn.* 2015;37(6):856–869.

59. Grossman D, White K, Hopkins K, Potter JE. The public health threat of anti-abortion legislation. *Contraception.* 2014;89(2):73.

60. Corley PC. Undue burden on women's right to seek an abortion: *Whole Woman's Health v. Hellerstedt. Just Sys J.* 2016;37(4):385–386.

61. Watts N, Adger WN, Agnolucci P, et al. Health and climate change: policy responses to protect public health. *Lancet.* 2015;386(10006):1861–1914.

62. Intergovernmental Panel on Climate Change. *Climate Change 2014: Mitigation of Climate Change.* Vol 3. New York, NY: Cambridge University Press; 2015.

63. Dunlap RE, McCright AM, Yarosh JH. The political divide on climate change: partisan polarization widens in the US. *Environment.* 2016;58(5):4–23.

64. Bloomberg Philanthropies Support LLC. America's Pledge Phase 1 Report: States, Cities, and Businesses in the United States Are Stepping Up on Climate Action. November 2017. Available at: https://www.americaspledgeonclimate.com. Accessed April 13, 2018.

65. Roser-Renouf C, Maibach EW Li J. Adapting to the changing climate: an assessment of local health department preparations for climate change-related health threats, 2008–2012. *PloS One.* 2016;11(3):e0151558.

66. Shultz JM, Kossin JP, Shepherd JM, et al. Risks, health consequences, and response challenges for small-island-based populations: observations from the 2017 Atlantic hurricane season. *Disaster Med Public Health Prep.* 2018:1–13.

67. Mays GP. Organization of the public health delivery system. In: Novick LF, Morrow CB, Mays GP, eds. *Public Health Administration: Principles for Population-Based Management.* 2nd ed. Sudbury, MA: Jones & Bartlett Learning;2008:83,87.

68. Centers for Medicare & Medicaid Services. National health care spending in 2016. Available at: https://www.cms.gov/Research-Statistics-Data-and-Systems/Statistics-Trends-and-Reports/ NationalHealthExpendData/Downloads/NHE-Presentation-Slides.pdf. Accessed February 20, 2018.

69. US National Library of Medicine. The Regional Medical Programs Collection. Available at: https://profiles.nlm.nih.gov/ps/retrieve/Narrative/RM/p-nid/94. Accessed April 14, 2018.

70. Melhado EM. Health planning in the United States and the decline of public-interest policy-making. *Milbank Q.* 2006;84(2):359–440.

71. National Conference of State Legislatures, CON – Certificate of Need State Laws. Available at: http://www.ncsl.org/research/health/con-certificate-of-need-state-laws.aspx. Accessed April 15, 2018.

72. US Department of Health and Human Services. Health IT legislation. Available at: https://www.healthit.gov/policy-researchers-implementers/health-it-legislation. Accessed April 15, 2018.

73. Centers for Disease Control and Prevention. Meaningful use. 2017. Available at: https://www.cdc.gov/ehrmeaningfuluse/introduction.html. Accessed April 15, 2018.

74. US Department of Health and Human Services. What is Medicare Part C? 2014. Available at: https://www.hhs.gov/answers/medicare-and-medicaid/what-is-medicare-part-c/index.html. Accessed March 6, 2018.

75. Lines L. The ACA vs. the doughnut hole: Medicare Part D utilization and costs. September 8, 2016. *The Medical Care Blog*. Available at: http://www.themedicalcareblog.com/aca_vs_doughnut_hole. Accessed March 6, 2018.

76. US Department of Veterans Affairs. Veterans Health Administration. Available at: https://www.va.gov/health. Accessed February 27, 2018.

77. US Department of Veterans Affairs. Veterans Choice Program frequently asked questions. Available at: http://www.triwest.com/en/veteran-services/veterans-choice-program-vcp/frequently-asked-questions. Accessed June 21, 2018.

78. US Department of Veterans Affairs. Veterans Access, Choice, and Accountability Act of 2014 Title I: Choice Program and Health Care Collaboration. Available at: https://www.va.gov/opa/choiceact/documents/choice-program-fact-sheet-final.pdf. Accessed February 27, 2018.

79. US Department of Veterans Affairs. 10 things about the Veterans Choice Program. Available at: https://www.va.gov/health/NewsFeatures/2017/July/Things-to-Know-About-the-Veteran-Choice-Program.asp. Accessed February 27, 2018.

80. US Department of Defense. TRICARE is changing, take command of your health. Available at: https://www.tricare.mil. Accessed February 27, 2018.

81. Centers for Disease Control and Prevention. *CDC's Policy Analytical Framework*. Atlanta, GA: US Department of Health and Human Services; 2013.

82. Jones J, Lee D, Bayhi L. The data-driven policy analysis framework as a template for healthcare policy analysis. *Ann Nurs Res Pract*. 2016;1(1):1005.

83. Weinick RM, Shin PW. *Monitoring the Health Care Safety Net: Developing Data-Driven Capabilities to Support Policy Making*. AHRQ Publication No. 04-0037. Rockville, MD: Agency for Healthcare Research and Quality; 2003.

84. Mays GP, Kennedy-Hendricks A. Organization of the public health system. In: Shi L, Johnson JA, eds. *Novick & Morrow's Public Health Administration: Principles for Population-Based Management*. 3rd ed. Burlington, MA: Jones & Bartlett Learning; 2014:86.

85. US Government Accountability Office. About GAO. Available at: https://www.gao.gov/about/index.html. Accessed February 27, 2018.

86. USA.gov. Budget of the United States Government. Available at: https://www.usa.gov/budget. Accessed February 27, 2018.

87. US Senate Committee on Appropriations. Committee jurisdiction. Available at: https://www.appropriations.senate.gov/about/jurisdiction. Accessed April 15, 2018.

88. US House of Representatives. Committee jurisdiction. Available at: https://waysandmeans.house.gov/committee-jurisdiction. Accessed April 16, 2018.

89. American Occupational Therapy Association. Key Senate and House Committees. Available at: https://www.aota.org/Conference-Events/Hill-Day/senate-house-committees.aspx. Accessed April 15, 2018.

90. US Food and Drug Administration. Compliance, enforcement & training. Available at: https://www.fda.gov/TobaccoProducts/GuidanceComplianceRegulatoryInformation/default.htm. Accessed March 6, 2018.

91. US Food and Drug Administration. Family Smoking Prevention and Tobacco Control Act—an overview. Available at: https://www.fda.gov/TobaccoProducts/Labeling/RulesRegulations Guidance/ucm246129.htm. Accessed March 6, 2018.

92. Gostin LO. Public health law. In: Novick LF, Morrow CB, Mays CB, eds. *Public Health Administration: Principles for Population-Based Management.* 2nd ed. Sudbury, MA: Jones & Bartlett Learning; 2008:135.

93. Merten PE. Do statewide planning and the consistency concept infringe on home rule authority? *J Plan Lit.* 1997;11(4):565–573.

10

Health Equity and Social Justice

Jaime A. Corvin, PhD, MSPH, CPH

INTRODUCTION

In the 20th century, after the epidemiologic transition that shifted focus from infectious diseases to chronic diseases, public health turned toward the role of social determinants of health and how social and ecological factors can influence health outcomes. A large body of evidence now points to the role of social factors in influencing health. The relationship, however, between these social factors and health is more complex than the infectious agent and disease relationship. A systems thinking approach is therefore required to understand and address the disparities faced by many. Addressing social determinants of health requires a deep look at all factors—from biology and genetics through global-level factors that require us to address deep-rooted political and structural factors that influence health.

This chapter will review the role of health equity and social justice in public health. It will provide a review of critical topics including the social–ecological factors that influence health and wellness. This chapter will highlight some of the prominent public health theories that help to guide our understanding of health and wellness. It will also guide you through reviewing the material and provide a case study to help you think critically about these concepts. In addition, some of these tasks have been covered in detail in previous chapters. By the end of this chapter, you should be able to apply the following tasks:

❑ Apply a social–ecological model to analyze population health issues.
❑ Design needs and resource assessments for communities or populations (covered in previous chapters).
❑ Assess how the values and perspectives of diverse individuals, communities, and cultures influence individual and society health behaviors, choices, and practices.
❑ Analyze the availability, acceptability, and accessibility of public health services and activities across diverse populations.
❑ Address health disparities in the delivery of public health services and activities.
❑ Use culturally appropriate concepts and skills to engage and empower diverse populations.
❑ Conduct culturally appropriate risk and resource assessment, management, and communication with individuals and populations (covered in previous chapters).

❑ Include representatives of diverse constituencies in partnerships.
❑ Incorporate strategies for interacting and collaborating with persons from diverse backgrounds.

MAJOR CONTENT

Because of advances in public health research, many major threats to health today are largely preventable.[1] A goal of public health professionals is to develop interventions to reduce preventable morbidity and mortality. To achieve this goal, emphasis has been placed on the social determinants of health and the conditions in which one lives. These issues are complex in nature and require a multifaceted approach to prevention and health promotion. As the field of public health works to address these issues, a keen understanding of the complex dynamics that influence health outcomes is required.

To begin to think about health equity and social justice, we must first define some key concepts and discuss the shift in public health toward addressing the root causes of health disparities in our nation and across the globe. This requires us to assess health disparities and necessitates the use of public health theories to guide the development of effective and efficient programs to combat these conditions. Ensuring that these programs and services are linguistically appropriate and culturally competent is vital to this goal.

What Is Population Health?

First, it is important to distinguish between population health—the mission of the field of public health—and individual health. The mission of public health is to "fulfill society's interest in assuring conditions in which people can be healthy."[2] To achieve this goal, public health researchers and practitioners take a population-based approach to understanding and addressing health outcomes. In fact, a hallmark of public health is the population-based focus. A population health focus requires an ecological approach to understanding factors that influence health and a systems approach to solving those problems. Grounded in a multidisciplinary approach, population health seeks to stabilize and improve health for all. This differs from an individual or conventional medicine approach. A public health approach requires collaboration across disciplines including medicine, nursing, nutrition, dentistry, social work, environmental sciences, health education, health services administration, and political advocacy, to name a few.[3] However, their activities focus on entire populations rather than on individual patients or clients. Examples of a population-based approach include the following[3]:

- Eradicating life-threatening diseases (e.g., measles, smallpox, polio) through the use of vaccinations
- Reducing death and disability attributable to unintentional injuries through policies designed to protect the safety of the public (e.g., bicycle helmet laws, seat belt laws)

- Assuring safe water
- Assuring a clean environment through the enforcement of regulatory controls and management of hazardous wastes
- Controlling and preventing infectious disease outbreaks
- Educating populations on health behaviors that put one at risk for chronic disease
- Facilitating community empowerment
- Assuring access to health services and care

Social Justice and Health Equity

A key cornerstone of the field of public health is its social justice approach to developing interventions with the goal of achieving health equity. **Social justice** is defined as "justice in terms of the distribution of wealth, opportunities, and privileges within a society."[4] Health equity is a term used by public health practitioners to describe the application of social justice principles to health.[5] **Health equity** was defined by US Department of Health and Human Services in *Healthy People 2020* as the "attainment of the highest level of health for all people."[6] Specifically, health equity relates to fairness, ensuring that no one is denied the opportunity to be healthy. As shown in Figure 10-1, health equity takes us a step beyond equality to ensuring that individuals have the resources needed to improve quality of life and health outcomes but that there is fairness in the allocation of these resources.[7] Health equity is providing fair opportunity, while eliminating gaps that exist between certain groups. To measure our progress in achieving public health's goal of health for all, we use **health disparities** as a metric. Reducing the gap in health disparities illustrates progress toward greater health equity.[5]

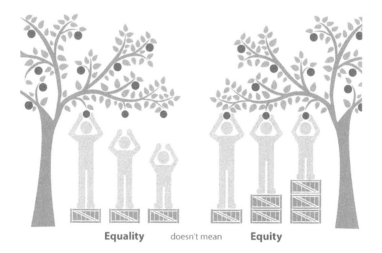

Equality   doesn't mean   **Equity**

Source: Neudorf et al.[7] Reprinted with permission from the Saskatoon Health Region; © 2014, Saskatoon Health Region.

Figure 10-1. Equality Doesn't Mean Equity

Health Disparities, Including Effects of Globalization on Health

To measure health disparities, we must employ a wide array of epidemiologic measures. Birth rates and infant mortality, as well as overall and cause-specific mortality rates, are useful measures for assessing this. We can drill deeper into incidence and prevalence rates for various disease conditions and how those conditions differ among subpopulations. For example, we might ask: Are women more at risk for a condition than men? Are African Americans more at risk for a condition than whites? Does socioeconomic status (SES) play a role? These epidemiologic measures help us to assess what is happening in our populations so that we can begin to address disparities. For more information on how to calculate standard epidemiologic measures, see Chapter 1, "Evidence-Based Approaches to Public Health."

Social Determinants of Health

The **social determinants of health** are factors in our social environment that contribute to or detract from health. Social determinants of health include but are not limited to SES, transportation, housing, and access to services, as well as discrimination by social grouping, or social or environmental stressors.

Research clearly illustrates how these factors play a significant role in adverse outcomes. For example, poverty limits access to healthy foods and SES is linked to safe neighborhoods. Social determinants can also provide protective effects. For example, we also know that education is a predictor of better health. Unfortunately, building interventions that address these social determinants is complicated. While extremely low-income communities are sometimes located adjacent to extremely wealthy communities, the resources are often strictly divided along invisible, rigid barriers that relegate individuals to the communities in which they were born and raised. This dichotomy of rich and poor, living virtually side by side, helps us to see the vast divide in the social determinants of health. Although seeing this dramatic difference in health outcomes and living conditions can be disheartening, it is not all bad news. Through application of our knowledge of the social determinants of health, we can improve individual and population health and advance health equity.[8–10]

Given the influence of social determinants on health, in 2011 the World Health Organization released a report titled *Realizing the Rio Political Declaration: Progress in Addressing the Social Determinants of Health*.[11] This report challenges countries around the globe to address the conditions in which we live, work, and age and how these conditions affect our health. There are five main themes from the Rio Declaration, which reflect a comprehensive public health approach to improving health and reducing disparities across populations[11]:

1. Adopt better governance for health and development.
2. Promote participation in policymaking and implementation.
3. Further orient the health sector toward reducing health inequities.

4. Strengthen global governance and collaboration.
5. Monitor progress and increase accountability.

This document serves as a global call to action to focus on good governance to ensure health for all. It iterates the government's responsibility to deliver health and to ensure that these services are equitably delivered. However, the responsibility of public health does not rest only with the government. Community participation is crucial for policy making and implementation. We all have a role to play to ensure health equity.

Cultural Competence

Cultural competence is one of the most effective ways to improve health equity and close the gap on health disparities. Cultural competence has been defined as "understanding and appropriately responding to the unique combination of cultural variables and the full range of dimensions of diversity that the professional and client/patient/ family bring to interactions."[12] Although public health has made incredible advancements in the past century, health disparities continue to plague populations nationally and globally, in part attributable to overlooking the significance of cultural competency in providing health care services.

Addressing Health Disparities by Applying Cultural Competency

One way to address cultural competency is by ensuring that health care services are provided in a culturally sensitive and linguistically appropriate manner. Doing so helps public health professionals improve health equity. Cultural competence promotes the need for programs and initiatives that meet people "where they are," with interventions that are linguistically appropriate and culturally sensitive. Public health leadership is now calling for culturally competent programs that do the following [13]:

- Embody the community voice, while garnering support and participation for long-term sustainability;
- Are inclusive of other strategies that also have the potential to influence the social determinants of health (e.g., housing, safety, education); and
- Ensure a platform for long-term sustainability and continuity of services from prevention to early detection, treatment, and evaluation.[13]

Importance of Public Health Theoretical Frameworks to Improve Health

To achieve the goal of reducing health disparities and to be effective, public health programs and interventions must provide gains in improving health, reducing the risk of disease, and assisting with managing illnesses. Public health programming is most effective when it addresses multiple systems-level factors (e.g., individual, organizational, and community). This is where public health theories are useful in informing public health programs and interventions.[14]

A theory presents a "systematic way of understanding events, behaviours, and/or situations."[15] Using a theoretical framework can help public health researchers better understand the disparities that exist among populations, especially among culturally and ethnically diverse groups. Many of the common health behavior theories used in public health can be applied to diverse cultural and ethnic groups, allowing public health practitioners to better understand their target populations, their differential risks for disease, and the opportunities for health promotion.[16]

Public health theories help shape and define the field. Although no single theory or conceptual framework dominates public health research or practice, several key theoretical frameworks exist. Key constructs from the most widely used theoretical models in health behavior are outlined as follows.

Health Belief Model

The **Health Belief Model** (HBM) "theorizes that people's beliefs about whether or not they are at risk for a disease or health problem, and their perceptions of the benefits of taking action to avoid it, influence their readiness to take action."[15] HBM was one of the first theories of health behavior, developed in the 1950s by a team from the US Public Health Service. The development of the HBM came about through trying to understand why individuals would not partake in tuberculosis screening. Core constructs encompass the following[14]:

- **Perceived susceptibility:** The individual's subjective assessment of his/her risk of developing the problem or condition.
- **Perceived severity:** The individual's assessment of the severity of a health problem and the potential consequences.
- **Perceived benefits:** The individual's assessment of the value of engaging in a health-promoting behavior to decrease risk of disease.
- **Perceived barriers:** The individual's perceptions of barriers that prevent health-promoting behaviors.
- **Cues to action:** Internal or external cues or triggers necessary to prompt engagement in health-promoting behaviors.
- **Self-efficacy:** The individual's perception of his/her ability to successfully perform the behavior.

The HBM is often applied for health concerns that are chronic and prevention-related and that have long asymptomatic stages. The model can be applied to conditions such as cancer through early cancer detection and cardiovascular disease through hypertension screening. The model is particularly beneficial for health conditions in which the individual's beliefs play an important role in guiding behaviors.

Transtheoretical Model and Stages of Change

The **Transtheoretical Model** (with the major construct—**Stages of Change**) was developed by Prochaska and DiClemente and posits that individuals move through six stages of change.[17] Changes in health behaviors require multiple actions and adaptations over time depending on the stage of change at which an individual is located. This model accounts for an individual's progression from not being ready to change through to the long-term maintenance of a healthful behavior. The notion of "readiness to change," or stage of change, has been widely examined in the public health behavior research and can be used to explain or predict behavior changes for smoking, physical activity, and eating habits, among others.[18] Figure 10-2 illustrates the first five steps of the Transtheoretical Model[17]:

1. **Precontemplation**: Individual has no intention of taking action now or in the foreseeable future (within the next 6 months).[17] Characterized by unawareness of the problematic nature of behaviors or their negative consequences.
2. **Contemplation**: Individual intends to engage in the healthy behavior at some point in foreseeable future (within the next 6 months). Characterized by recognition that the behavior is problematic.
3. **Preparation (determination)**: Individual is ready to act and plans to engage in the behavior within the next 30 days. Characterized by taking small steps toward the behavior change.
4. **Action**: Individual recently changed his/her behavior (within the last 6 months) and plans to continue the behavior change. Individuals may exhibit this by modifying their problem behavior or acquiring new healthy behaviors.
5. **Maintenance**: Individual has sustained his/her behavior change (more than 6 months). Characterized by intent to maintain the behavior change. Focus of this stage is to prevent relapse to earlier stages.
6. **Termination**: Individual has no desire to return to the unhealthy behaviors, and relapse is unlikely. This stage is rarely considered in health promotion programs, and individuals are most often regarded as staying in the maintenance stage.[17,18]

The Stages of Change are useful, for example, to incite behavior change among people at high risk for diabetes or to improve the success of health counseling.

Social Cognitive Theory

Social Cognitive Theory (SCT), based on Bandura's Social Learning Theory, posits that learning occurs in a social context with a dynamic and reciprocal integration of the person,

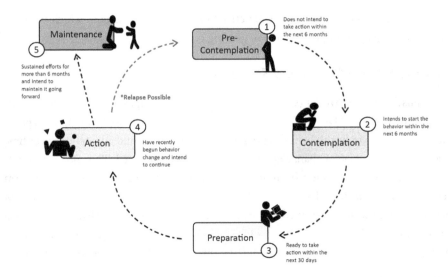

Figure 10-2. The Steps of the Transtheoretical Model

environment, and behavior.[19] SCT emphasizes social influence and external and internal social reinforcement. Unlike some other health promotion theories, SCT focuses on the maintenance of behavior rather than on just the initiation of healthy behaviors. SCT is based on the belief that people learn through their own experiences but also by observing the actions of others and the results of those actions. The basic tenets of SCT include the following[19]:

- **Reciprocal determinism**: Refers to the dynamic and reciprocal interaction of person, environment, and behavior.
- **Behavioral capability**: An individual's ability to perform a behavior through essential knowledge and skills.
- **Observational learning**: The ability to witness and observe a behavior conducted by others and model or reproduce those actions.
- **Reinforcements**: Refers to the internal or external responses to a person's behavior that affect the likelihood of continuing or discontinuing the behavior. Reinforcements can be positive or negative.
- **Expectations**: Anticipated consequences of an individual's behavior. Expectations derive largely from previous experience.
- **Self-efficacy**: An individual's confidence in his/her ability to successfully perform a behavior.

Theory of Planned Behavior

Theory of Planned Behavior (TPB), which grew out of the Theory of Reasoned Action,[20] was proposed by Icek Ajzen in 1985[21] to explain and predict how a behavior is formed.

Critical to this model is behavioral intent and the belief that these intentions are influenced by the likelihood that the behavior will result in an expected outcome, as well as the subjective evaluation of the risks and benefits of such outcomes. The TPB posits that behavioral achievement is dependent upon both intention (motivation) and behavioral control. The TPB is comprised of six constructs, representing an individual's control over a behavior:

1. **Attitude toward act or behavior**: Belief that a certain behavior or act will make a positive or negative contribution.
2. **Behavioral intention**: Motivational factors that influence a behavior; the stronger the intention to perform the behavior, the more likely an individual will perform the behavior.
3. **Subjective norm:** Factors around the individual (e.g., social network, cultural norms, group belief) and the individual's belief as to whether others will approve or disapprove of their behavior.
4. **Social norms:** Considers what is normative in a group.
5. **Perceived power:** Perceived factors that act as barriers or facilitators to the behavior.
6. **Perceived behavioral control:** Individual's belief of how easy or hard it is to adopt a certain behavior.

The TPB has been used to predict health behaviors including substance use, breastfeeding, and health services utilization. However, the theory is not without limitations as it does not account for environmental and economic influences that play an important role in the adoption of health behaviors.[14,16]

Rogers's Diffusion of Innovations

Diffusion of innovation was proposed by Everett Rogers, a communication theorist and sociologist, in 1995. Diffusion of innovations explains how innovation (e.g., an idea, behavior, or product) gains momentum and spreads throughout a population. In public health, adoption of new behaviors or beliefs or products is a process that takes time as some individuals are more likely to adopt a new behavior than others. Thus, it is imperative to understand the target audience when promoting the adoption of new behaviors. Specifically, there are five adopter categories[14,16]:

1. **Innovators:** Those individuals who are the first to try and adopt new innovation.
2. **Early adopters:** Those who embrace change. They are typically leaders who are aware of a need for change and are comfortable with new ideas.
3. **Early majority:** Those individuals who adopt new ideas before the majority.
4. **Late majority:** Those individuals skeptical of change who will adopt only after the majority.
5. **Laggards**: Those individuals who are very skeptical of change.

See Figure 10-3[14] for examples of how the population typically moves toward innovation.

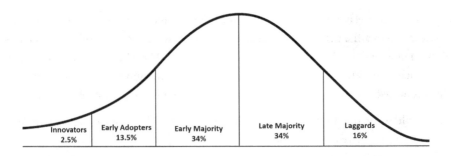

Figure 10-3. Diffusions of Innovation Theory

Social-Ecological Model

Traditionally, health promotion has targeted individual-level factors such as knowledge, beliefs, and skills for behavior change. However, as ecological and systems thinking become more prominent, programs and interventions have taken a broader approach to target other levels of influence, such as policy-level, community, and organizational-level factors. The **Social–Ecological Model** (SEM) was developed to understand this complex, multifaceted, and dynamic relationship between an individual and the environmental factors that influence health behaviors and health outcomes. These concepts, introduced in the 1970s and formalized by Bronfenbrenner,[22] have evolved over time. SEM is a systems model with multiple bands of influence in which each band represents one of the five hierarchical levels of the model: (1) **individual,** (2) **interpersonal,** (3) **organizational,** (4) **community,** and (5) **policy,** as outlined in Figure 10-4.[23]

The SEM model allows public health researchers to understand risk and protective factors and to address leverage points for health promotion and prevention. For example, if we seek to address obesity, we must look at various levels of influence that will have an impact on the outcome. Physical activity is influenced by self-efficacy at the individual level, social support and the role of family and friends at the interpersonal level, and perceptions of crime and safety that influence one's ability to exercise outside at the community level. Workplaces and schools also play a role at the organizational level as do local, state, and national policies related to nutrition and healthy eating at the policy level.

Practice Questions

Vignette 1: *Esperanza is a 35-year-old woman living in an area known as Villa Miseria, an overcrowded slum near Buenos Aires, Argentina. There is no sanitation system and the electrical power is not always consistent. Approximately a mile away is the vibrant city of Buenos Aires. The health and economic disparities between these two areas is glaring. Esperanza does not have access to the same services as a mother living in Buenos Aires and is 35% more likely to die in childbirth than a mother in Buenos Aires.*

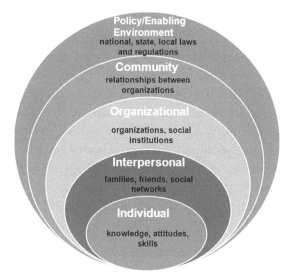

Source: Adapted from Centers for Disease Control and Prevention.[23]

Figure 10-4. The Social–Ecological Model: A Framework for Prevention

1. To improve health outcomes in Villa Miseria, which of the following principles would be helpful?
   a. Health determinism
   b. Social justice
   c. Epidemiologic studies
   d. The Transtheoretical Model

Answer: b. Social justice embodies principles of equity and access for all. Addressing these inequities can help to improve health and ensure access for those in need. Other choices do not directly apply.

2. The single best predictor of poor health in Esperanza's community, as well as in society in general, is
   a. Poverty
   b. Race
   c. Religion
   d. Gender

Answer: a. The single best indicator of health is one's SES, which is tied closely to class. Simply, those at the top have more and better access to resources, more power and control, and, on average, live longer, healthier lives. Although other responses are important, the single best predictor is poverty.[24]

3. A public health team was interested in assisting in Villa Miseria to address concerns about water and sanitation. They seek to do so in a culturally appropriate way. Which of the following is the best example of culturally appropriate community engagement and empowerment strategies?
   a. Providing health services and implementing programs that have proven to be successful in communities that are culturally distinct from the focus community
   b. Avoiding bias by developing programs before meeting with community leaders and investigating the specific needs of the community
   c. Choosing interventions that have previously been applied in the community by local and national political leaders
   d. Implementing health projects that result in the reciprocal transfer of knowledge and skills among all collaborators and partners

Answer: d. Implementing health projects that result in the reciprocal transfer of knowledge and skills among all collaborators and partners is imperative to ensure success and sustainability. This places the community in a position of power, where their voices are being heard. While including community partners and implementing programs with a proven track record is important, simply translating the language is not enough. In addition, the community should always be included in every step of development and implementation to ensure success.

4. A stakeholder in the proposed water and sanitation program is best described as
   a. Anyone involved in the operations or affected by the program in Villa Miseria
   b. The beneficiaries and participants in the program in Villa Miseria
   c. The sponsors and administrators of the program in Villa Miseria
   d. The financial investors in the program in Villa Miseria

Answer: a. Stakeholders can be anyone involved with or affected by a program. This may include the recipients of the program, the surrounding communities, the providers involved, and those who operate the program.

5. The biological, environmental, behavioral, organizational, political, and social factors that are contributing to health in Villa Miseria are commonly referred to as
   a. Social justice
   b. Determinants of health
   c. Health behaviors
   d. Causal factors

Answer: b. The biological, environmental, behavioral, organizational, political, and social factors are referred to as determinants of health. Other choices do not directly apply.

Vignette 2: *A health educator gives a presentation on distracted driving. Following her presentation, she discusses distracted driving with a student who just lost a loved one in a distracted driving crash. The student still texts and drives but is asking for advice and assistance in how to change these behaviors.*

6. According to the Transtheoretical Model, the student is in what stage?
   a. Contemplation
   b. Preparation
   c. Action
   d. Maintenance

Answer: b. The student is ready to take action. This is characterized by her small steps toward the behavior change, including sharing her story and asking advice of the health educator.

7. As the health educator engages students further, she finds that many students currently text while driving and do not see the relationship between texting and car crashes. For students at the precontemplation stage of change, the health educator would most likely attempt to
   a. Encourage their behaviors and actions
   b. Develop cues that help to remind individuals not to use their phone while driving
   c. Share testimonials from those who have lost a loved one in a distracted driving event
   d. Provide training and guidance to prevent relapse behavior

Answer: c. Individuals in the precontemplation stage are still largely unaware or unwilling to admit there is a problem. The first step is to attempt to increase their perceptions that texting and driving is a problem. One way to do this is to expose them to data and testimonials that highlight the problem.

8. Which of the following is characteristic of a health care system based on social justice?
   a. A distribution of resources that removes human biases by allowing the market to decide how they are allocated
   b. An individual's ability to pay is considered inconsequential to receiving medical care
   c. A single-payer health care system
   d. A system in which the recipients of health care determine how resources should be allocated

Answer: b. Ensuring that individuals receive care, regardless of ability to pay, is a central component of social justice. Other choices do not apply in terms of defining social justice.

9. Which of the following models explains the relationship between SES and health by illustrating that health status and social standing are linked to a combination of interrelated social, cultural, psychological, and environmental factors?
   a. Transtheoretical Model
   b. Social Learning Model

c. Social–Ecological Model

d. Theory of Reasoned Action

Answer: c. The SEM evaluates the interrelated set of factors that influence health and takes a systems approach to understanding factors that influence health.

CONCLUSION

Over the past century, public health has made leaps and bounds with reducing mortality and morbidity of infectious diseases, providing public services, and increasing the longevity of individuals across the globe. Public health professionals have noted a stagnation of improvements in recent years, mostly attributable to health disparities across populations in which many subgroups still perform poorly by various health indices. Social justice and health equity have become core concepts in the pursuit of providing quality health to all members of society. Pursuing these goals is supported through collecting data and analyzing results with epidemiologic measures, by addressing the various social determinants of health, and also by building interventions based on various theoretical frameworks, such as the Transtheoretical Model, the HBM, the SEM, and the SCT. These interventions are also assisted by ensuring cultural competency among health care providers so that health care is provided in a manner that is appropriate for the recipients.

REFERENCES

1. World Health Organization. Global health risks: mortality and burden of disease attributable to selected major risks. 2009. Available at: http://www.who.int/healthinfo/global_burden_disease/GlobalHealthRisks_report_full.pdf. Accessed November 17, 2017.

2. Institute of Medicine. *The Future of Public Health*. Washington, DC: The National Academies Press; 1988.

3. American Public Health Association. What is public health? Available at: https://www.apha.org/what-is-public-health. Accessed March 21, 2018.

4. Social justice. English Oxford Living Dictionaries. Available at: https://en.oxforddictionaries.com/definition/social_justice. Accessed March 21, 2018.

5. Braveman P. What are health disparities and health equity? We need to be clear. *Public Health Rep*. 2014;129(suppl 2):5–8.

6. Healthy People 2020. Disparities. US Department of Health and Human Services. Available at: https://www.healthypeople.gov/2020/about/foundation-health-measures/Disparities#5. Accessed March 21, 2018.

7. Neudorf C, Kryzanowski J, Turner H, et al. Better Health for All Series 3: Advancing Health Equity in Health Care. Saskatoon, SK: Saskatoon Health Region. 2014. Available at: https://www.saskatoonhealthregion.ca/locations_services/Services/Health-Observatory/Documents/Reports-Publications/2014_shr_phase3_advancing_healthequity_healthcare_series.pdf. Accessed June 27, 2018.

8. Healthy People 2020. Social determinants of health. US Department of Health and Human Services. Available at: https://www.healthypeople.gov/2020/topics-objectives/topic/social-determinants-of-health. Accessed March 21, 2018.

9. Adler NE, Newman K. Socioeconomic disparities in health: pathways and policies inequality. *Health Aff (Millwood)*. 2002;21(2):60–76.

10. Walker RE, Keane CR, Burke JG. Disparities and access to healthy food in the United States: a review of food deserts literature. *Health Place*. 2010;16(5):876–884.

11. World Conference on Social Determinants of Health. Rio political declaration on social determinants of health. World Health Organization. 2011. Available at: http://www.who.int/sdhconference/declaration/Rio_political_declaration.pdf?ua=1. Accessed November 17, 2017.

12. American Speech-Language-Hearing Association. Cultural competence. Available at: http://www.asha.org/Practice-Portal/Professional-Issues/Cultural-Competence. Accessed March 21, 2018.

13. Horowitz C, Lawlor EF. Appendix D Community approaches to addressing health disparities. Institute of Medicine. 2008. Available at: https://www.ncbi.nlm.nih.gov/books/NBK215366. Accessed September 9, 2018.

14. Glanz K, Rimer BK, Viswanath K. *Health Behavior: Theory, Research, and Practice*. 5th ed. San Francisco, CA: Jossey-Bass; 2015.

15. Glanz K. Social and behavioral theories. Available at: https://obssr.od.nih.gov/wp-content/uploads/2016/05/Social-and-Behavioral-Theories.pdf. Accessed May 3, 2018.

16. National Cancer Institute. Theory at a glance: a guide for health promotion practice. US Department of Health and Human Services. 2005. Available at: https://www.sbccimplementationkits.org/demandrmnch/wp-content/uploads/2014/02/Theory-at-a-Glance-A-Guide-For-Health-Promotion-Practice.pdf. Accessed November 17, 2017.

17. Prochaska JO, DiClemente CC. Stages and processes of self-change of smoking: toward an integrative model of change. *J Consult Clin Psychol*. 1983;51(3):390–395.

18. Prochaska JO, DiClemente CC. Transtheoretical therapy: toward a more integrative model of change. *Psychother Theory Res Pract*. 1982;19(3):276–288.

19. Boston University School of Public Health. The Social Cognitive Theory. Available at: http://sphweb.bumc.bu.edu/otlt/MPH-Modules/SB/BehavioralChangeTheories/BehavioralChangeTheories5.html. Accessed May 3, 2018.

20. Fishbein M, Ajzen I. *Belief, Attitude, Intention, and Behavior: An Introduction to Theory and Research*. Reading, MA: Addison-Wesley; 1975.

21. Ajzen I. From intentions to actions: a theory of planned behavior. In: Kuhl J, Beckmann J, eds. *Action Control: From Cognition to Behavior.* 1st ed. Berlin, Germany: Springer-Verlag Berlin Heidelberg; 1985:11–39.

22. Bronfenbrenner U. Ecological systems theory. In: Vasta R, ed. *Six Theories of Child Development: Revised Formulations and Current Issues.* London, England: Jessica Kingsley Publishers; 1992:187–249.

23. Centers for Disease Control and Prevention. The social-ecological model: a framework for prevention. Available at: https://www.cdc.gov/violenceprevention/overview/social-ecologicalmodel.html. Accessed April 21, 2018.

24. Adler NE. Reaching for a healthier life: facts on socioeconomic status and health in the US. 2007. The John D. and Catherine T. MacArthur Foundation Research Network on Socioeconomic Status and Health. Available at: http://www.macses.ucsf.edu/downloads/reaching_for_a_healthier_life.pdf. Accessed November 17, 2017.

Contributors

EDITORS

Karen D. Liller, PhD, CPH, is a Professor at the University of South Florida College of Public Health, specializing in public health and injury prevention. Dr. Liller holds undergraduate and graduate degrees in medical technology, technical education, and education (curriculum and instruction) with a cognate area of public health. She has held numerous administrative positions including Associate Dean for Academics and Student Affairs at the College of Public Health, Dean of the University of South Florida Graduate School, and Associate Vice President for Research and Innovation. Dr. Liller is presently the Director of the Activist Lab at the College and the Strategic Lead for the area of policy, practice, and leadership. She also is an established Reviewer and Item Writer for the Certified Public Health exam. (Chapters 5 and 7)

Jaime A. Corvin, PhD, MSPH, CPH, is an Associate Professor at the University of South Florida College of Public Health. She joined the College in 2006. Trained in community and family health and social and behavioral sciences, Dr. Corvin's areas of research include global maternal and child health issues, global health disparities, and chronic disease management. Dr. Corvin leads the development and implementation of the integrated core at the College. She has both written and reviewed questions for the Certified Public Health exam and has served on numerous panels about the role of the Certified Public Health exam in the future of public health education. (Chapters 5 and 10)

ASSOCIATE EDITOR

Hari H. Venkatachalam, MPH, CPH, is a graduate of the University of South Florida College of Public Health where he concentrated in epidemiology and global communicable diseases. Mr. Venkatachalam has undergraduate degrees in biological sciences, neuroscience, and religious studies, as well as graduate certificates in biostatistics and infection control. He has worked internationally under Dr. David Simmons at Western Sydney University on the social determinants of diabetes. Mr. Venkatachalam also served as a Teaching Assistant for the integrated core courses at the University of South Florida and was responsible for leading analysis labs. (Chapters 1 and 5)

AUTHORS

Amy Alman, PhD, is an Associate Professor at the University of South Florida College of Public Health. Her current research interests include the epidemiology of diabetes and cardiovascular disease, particularly the moderating and mediating roles of adiposity, inflammation, and infections. (Chapter 5)

Chighaf Bakour, MD, PhD, MPH, CPH, is a Visiting Assistant Professor at the University of South Florida College of Public Health. Her research interests include maternal and child health and chronic diseases, particularly the role of sleep duration in adolescents and young adults as a risk factor for chronic diseases. (Chapter 1)

Alicia Best, PhD, is an Assistant Professor at the University of South Florida College of Public Health. She is a Sociobehavioral Researcher and a Certified Health Education Specialist with academic training and experience in health education and promotion, health communications, and cancer-related health disparities. (Chapter 2)

Pamela C. Birriel, PhD, MPH, CHES, completed her doctoral training in public health with a concentration in crosscultural and community-based research, design, and evaluation. Her passion in the field stems from her drive to help underserved and vulnerable populations through culturally and linguistically tailored health education programs. She is currently completing a fellowship focusing on cancer genomics health communications. (Chapter 6)

Katherine Drabiak, JD, is an Assistant Professor at the University of South Florida College of Public Health and is Codirector of the Law & Medicine Scholarly Concentration Program at Morsani College of Medicine. Dr. Drabiak focuses her teaching and research in health care law, public health law, and law and policy relating to emerging technology. (Chapter 4)

Barbara Langland-Orban, PhD, is a Professor at the University of South Florida College of Public Health. She specializes in hospital management, quality management, accreditation and licensing, medical staff affairs, and strategic and business planning. Dr. Orban was a Faculty Member in health services administration at the University of Florida from 1985 to 1997 where she served terms as Department Chair and Program Director of the nationally ranked Graduate Program in Health and Hospital Administration. (Chapter 9)

Jennifer Marshall, PhD, CPH, is an Assistant Professor at the University of South Florida College of Public Health and the Lead Evaluator for Florida's Maternal, Infant, and Early Childhood Home Visiting and Early Childhood Comprehensive Systems initiatives. She conducts community-based research assessing infant mortality prevention programs, family-centered care and access to medical and developmental services, and infant mental health community initiatives. Her research interests stem from over 25 years of experience working with community-based programs as a Practitioner, Program Director, and Researcher. (Chapters 6 and 7)

Dinorah Martinez Tyson, PhD, is an Assistant Professor at the University of South Florida College of Public Health and a Courtesy Professor in anthropology. She has extensive experience in qualitative methods and in community engaged research. She has worked closely with various community organizations to address health disparities among ethnic minorities and underserved populations in the Tampa Bay area and Spanish-speaking Caribbean. Her community experience has also provided her with invaluable insights about partnership and coalition building processes. (Chapter 6)

Steven Mlynarek, PhD, is a Professor at the University of South Florida College of Public Health. His current research areas include exposure assessment, aerosol technology, and indoor environmental quality. He has obtained professional certification as a Qualified Environmental Professional and is a Certified Industrial Hygienist. (Chapter 5)

Kathleen O'Rourke, PhD, CPH, is a Professor Emeritus at the University of South Florida College of Public Health. She has served as the Location Lead Investigator for two sites of the National Children's Study: Hillsborough County and Orange County, Florida. Her research focus expands upon her interests in developing and evaluating programs that can address maternal and child health disparities among minority populations within community-based settings. She has conducted a number of maternal and child health research projects on the US/Mexico border and is currently evaluating the relationship of post-traumatic stress disorder and reproductive outcomes among women in the military. (Chapter 1)

Claudia Parvanta, PhD, is a Professor at the University of South Florida College of Public Health and the Director of, as well as a Professor at, the Florida Prevention Research Center. Dr. Parvanta's expertise lies in social marketing, communication, and health literacy. In Philadelphia, she researched and contributed to projects to improve health literacy in the city's public health centers, to increase colorectal cancer screening among minorities, and to train health professions students in culturally competent communication. (Chapter 2)

Donna J. Petersen, ScD, MHS, CPH, is Dean of the College of Public Health at the University of South Florida and Senior Associate Vice President, University of South Florida Health. She is Editor Emerita of the Maternal and Child Health Journal, Founding Member and Past President of the National Board of Public Health Examiners, Immediate Past Chair of the Council on Education for Public Health, and Chair of the Association of Schools and Programs of Public Health. From 2011 to 2015, she chaired the Association of Schools and Programs of Public Health–sponsored task force, Framing the Future: The Second Hundred Years of Education in Public Health. She is on the Tampa Bay

Partnership's OneBay Healthy Communities Executive Committee, the Hillsborough County Health Care Advisory Board, the Foundation for a Healthy St. Petersburg Board, and the Board of Trustees of the Tampa Preparatory School. Among her many honors, she was named Distinguished Alumna in 2011 by The Johns Hopkins University. (Chapter 3)

Sandra Potthoff, PhD, is a Professor at the University of South Florida College of Public Health. She was previously a Faculty Member at the University of Minnesota where she served as the Director of the Master of Healthcare Administration Program for eight years. Her current research entails studying hospital collaboration strategies for population health management and the adoption and implementation of the Baldrige Performance Excellence Framework for cross-sector community collaboratives. (Chapter 8)

Vijay Prajapati, BDS, CPH, is an MPH student at the University of South Florida College of Public Health, concentrating in epidemiology. He acquired his BDS from Gujarat University, India in 2016. He is a member of the Florida Prevention Research Center contributing to increasing screening for colorectal cancer in Florida. (Chapter 2)

Zachary Pruitt, PhD, MHA, CPH, is an Assistant Professor at the University South Florida College of Public Health. Prior to academics, Dr. Pruitt directed policy and operations for managed care organizations. His research interests include the examination of health care costs, quality, and access among those insured by Medicaid, health care management applications, patient navigator programs, and the integration of medical and social care for vulnerable populations. (Chapter 4)

Troy Quast, PhD, is an Associate Professor at the University of South Florida College of Public Health. His research interests include the impact of economic conditions on health status, Medicaid policy, and the impact of natural disasters on health status and the utilization of health services. He has been awarded research funding by the National Institutes of Health to examine the treatment of children displaced after Hurricane Katrina and has an interest in using large data sets for analysis of population health issues. (Chapter 1)

Rema Ramakrishnan, PhD, has experience in clinical pediatrics in India and extensive training in public health, including community-based research, evaluation, and advanced epidemiological and biostatistical methods. Her research interest is in reproductive, perinatal, and environmental epidemiology. (Chapter 6)

Ira Richards, PhD, is a Professor at the University of South Florida College of Public Health. His research interests encompass petrochemical and agrochemical industries, manufacturing, the workplace, and general industrial and environmental issues, as well as a wide range of classes of chemicals including pesticides, solvents, heavy metals, irritants, particulates, carcinogens, pharmaceuticals, and illicit substances. His current research focuses on respiratory irritants and the expression of biomarkers of inflammation and oxidative stress from exposures to chemical agents. (Chapter 5)

William M. Sappenfield, MD, MPH, CPH, is a Professor at the University of South Florida College of Public Health. Prior to academics, Dr. Sappenfield served as a Maternal and Child Health Epidemiologist at the Centers for Disease Control and Prevention, in state public health agencies, and for CityMatCH; he ultimately served as a Lead of Centers for Disease Control and Prevention's Maternal and Child Health Epidemiology Program. Currently, he also serves as Director of The Chiles Center and the Florida Perinatal Quality Collaborative where he uses epidemiology, research, public health practice and quality improvement sciences to improve the health of women, children, and families especially in the perinatal period. (Chapter 6)

Anna Torrens Armstrong, PhD, CPH, is an Assistant Professor at the University of South Florida College of Public Health. She teaches courses in the undergraduate health education minor track. Her research interests include teaching innovation, school-based health services, developmental evaluation and design thinking, collective impact initiatives, military health promotion, and resiliency. Anna also serves as an Adjunct Faculty (online) at the Johns Hopkins Krieger School of Arts and Sciences Advanced Academic Program in the Department of Communication. (Chapter 7)

Thomas Unnasch, PhD, is a Distinguished Health Professor at the University of South Florida College of Public Health. His research has focused upon vector-borne diseases and the human filarial infections. His laboratory research concentrates on areas that have a direct impact on disease control and elimination programs targeting vector-borne pathogens worldwide. (Chapter 5)

Wei Wang, PhD, is an Associate Professor at the University of South Florida College of Public Health. Dr. Wang has been involved as the Leading Statistician in multiple prevention trails, including classroom and family-based programs focused on reducing substance use and increasing academic performance. He has been a long-term member of the Prevention Science & Methodology Group and currently serves as the University of South Florida Subcontract Personal Investigator for three federal funded grants. (Chapter 1)

Jacqueline Wiltshire, PhD, is an Assistant Professor at the University of South Florida College of Public Health. She is a Health Services Researcher, focusing on women's health, aging, and racial/ethnic disparities in health care utilization and outcomes. Dr. Wiltshire has published research on race/ethnicity and socioeconomic status in access to medical care, trust in physicians, patient engagement in care, health information use, and affordability of care. (Chapter 9)

Janice Zgibor, PhD, is an Associate Professor at the University of South Florida College of Public Health and Director of the DrPH Program. Dr. Zgibor is a Coinvestigator on a study called MOVE UP, which is a translation of the Look AHEAD study. This intervention is a community-based trial examining the impact of this intervention on weight loss and physical function in older adults using community health workers to deliver the intervention. Dr. Zgibor recently completed a cluster-randomized trial in primary care entitled Redesigning Medication Intensification Effectiveness for Diabetes. (Chapter 1)

Index